PREFACE

This laboratory manual is the Sixth Edition of one designed to provide a source of instructional procedures for use in teaching the laboratory aspects of immunology. Many of the ideas contained herein were originated by our immunology mentor, the late Matt Dodd of The Ohio State University. Dr. Dodd, a recipient of the American Society of Microbiology's Carski Foundation Distinguished Teaching Award, exerted a profound influence on the immunological training of students for over 30 years. It is to him that this continuing effort is dedicated.

The text of the manual has been kept to a minimum to allow flexible use of it with any of a number of excellent textbooks available today. The directions and experimental design have been kept as simple as possible for clarity and ease of completion within normal laboratory periods. It is emphasized that these experiments are designed for instructional purposes and are not intended to be necessarily used for research, which is beyond the scope of this manual.

As before, we have endeavored to provide detailed, supplementary instructions for preparation of reagents and equipment to assist the instructors. This includes listing sources of supply for less common materials. We have incorporated commercial reagents in a few of the experiments for convenience, but our selection does not necessarily constitute an endorsement of that product.

The science of immunology has grown remarkably in the last 20 years, especially in the area of cellular immunology. Although we have tried to include a number of experiments reflecting this modern emphasis, we were limited in selection due to the time required for completion of many of them, their need for specialized equipment, and other factors detracting from their suitability as classroom experiments. The entire manual has been updated, and many new experiments have been added. Yet, we have retained those experiments that have been proven especially useful in the past and continue to serve the basic needs of the modern laboratory.

We are grateful for the constructive criticisms of many students and instructors, especially those from Dr. Virginia C. Kelley, Auburn University. Any mistakes that may be encountered are those of the authors, and we continue to be receptive to your comments.

CONTENTS

Section I
BASIC IMMUNOLOGY

Exercise 1

THE USE OF SEROLOGICAL GLASSWARE

The following experiments are designed to acquaint the beginning student with fundamental principles and techniques of serological laboratory work.

1. Titration of a Surface Active Agent—Doubling Dilutions

The purpose of this experiment is to illustrate what is meant by the titration of a substance. A titration is the estimation of the activity or content of a reagent. Although sera are not used in this experiment, the same general method is often used in measuring antibody content of sera. Usually, doubling, or $\log_2$, dilutions are made when titering a serum.

Since this technique gives only a crude approximation of the strength of the reagent being titrated, it is important to use careful technique. Customarily, titrations employ doubling dilutions and hence the result may vary from 50% to 100%. If the same pipette is used throughout the titration, an error in "carry over" is likely to occur. In spite of these limitations, the doubling dilution technique is widely used when only an estimate of strength is desired.

This experiment also demonstrates lysis of erythrocytes in isotonic solutions. Many substances have this lytic capacity (e.g., surface active agents, certain organic solvents, toxins, and enzymes). Since serological glassware is frequently cleaned with detergents or chromic acid, both of which are very hemolytic, thorough rinsing after such cleaning is indicated. For this experiment, hemolysis is demonstrated with saponin, a plant glycoside, commonly used as a foaming agent.

PROCEDURE

1. Set up a series of ten serological tubes in a rack.

2. Add 0.5 ml physiological saline to tubes 2 through 10.

3. Add 0.5 ml 0.1% saponin to tubes 1 and 2.

4. Mix the contents of tube 2 thoroughly and transfer 0.5 ml to tube 3; mix and transfer 0.5 ml to tube 4; and so on through tube 9.

5. Add 0.5 ml 2% erythrocytes to each tube.

6. Mix and incubate in a 37°C water bath for 30 min, then centrifuge at 1500 x g for 3 min.

7. Record hemolysis on the basis of +, 2+, 3+, and 4+.

8. The titer is the highest dilution of reagent that gives any evidence of the desired reaction.

    Titer: _____

2. Titration of a Precipitinogen—Log Dilutions

Reagents that possess extremely high activity over a broad range of dilutions are often titered in tenfold, or log_{10}, dilutions. This procedure is subject to even more error than in doubling dilutions, and more care must be taken in its preparation. In this procedure, the pipettes are discarded after each transfer and before mixing. Occasionally, when the endpoint is found to be between two tenfold dilutions, it is helpful to prepare a second titration by the doubling dilution method between these two points in order to find the titer more exactly.

Tenfold dilutions are commonly used to enumerate populations of bacteria or viruses, to determine the effectiveness of antibiotics, or to determine the percipitating range of soluble antigens (precipitinogen).

PROCEDURE

1. By means of a capillary pipette, introduce into the bottoms of seven small-bore (5-mm I.D.) test tubes a constant amount of anti-~~bovine~~ *turkey* serum, the exact quantity not being critical.

2. In a separate set of six conventional serological tubes, prepare tenfold dilutions of the homologous antigen (place 0.9 ml saline in each tube; add 0.1 ml antigen to tube 1, discard pipette; mix with new pipette and transfer 0.1 ml to tube 2, discard pipette; etc.). *Discard* 0.1 ml after mixing contents of tube 6.

3. Starting with the highest dilution, transfer a small amount of antigen to a serum tube with a capillary pipette so that the antigen forms a layer over the antiserum. Do not mix.

4. Proceed to the next dilution and so on until all dilutions have been layered over respective aliquots of antiserum. Layer a like amount of saline over antiserum for a control.

5. Incubate the tubes for an hour at room temperature, making observations every 15 min.

6. Record the greatest dilution of antigen that the antiserum is capable of detecting: _____.

3. Use of Microtiter Equipment

In practice, gross dilutions with pipettes have often been replaced by special equipment designed to speed up the process and to economize the amount of reagents needed for standard titrations. The principle is exactly the same, but the equipment is quite different. Plastic trays with indented wells are used in place of serologic tubes and calibrated, metal transfer diluters are substituted for pipettes. Titrations are commonly performed in 25 or 50 μl quantities.

PROCEDURE

1. Dispense 50 μl saline in wells 2 through 10 in one row of a microtiter tray, using a calibrated pipette dropper or a micropipette (usage will be demonstrated). Place an equal amount in well 1 as a control.

2. Using a similar dispenser, add 50 μl 1/10 anti-sheep RBC serum to wells 1 and 2.

3. Mix the contents of well 2 with a 50 μl calibrated microdiluter by twisting the handle back and forth with your fingers.

4. Carefully transfer the microdiluter to well 3 and repeat mixing motion.

5. Continue through well 10. Clean dispensers and microdiluters as directed.

6. Dispense 25 μl 2% sheep RBCs into all wells. Mix by vibration.

7. Allow the tray to stand until RBCs settle out, then read agglutination by pattern. Nonagglutinated cells will settle out in "buttons" with smooth edges while agglutinated buttons will be ragged.

Exercise 2

PREPARATION OF IMMUNIZING AGENTS

Suspensions of microorganisms employed for artificial active immunization are referred to as vaccines. Such preparations usually contain several different antigens. Other immunizing agents such as erythrocyte suspensions and protein solutions are also used for certain types of artificial active immunization.

Each student or group of students, as assigned, will be responsible for the preparation of at least one immunizing agent, the immunization of a suitable animal with that agent, and the standardization of the resulting antiserum.

1. Bacterial Vaccines

An effective vaccine must be specific (i.e., it must contain the antigens that will stimulate the production of protective antibodies). It must also be made safe by rendering the substances nontoxic or avirulent in immunizing doses. Thus, most vaccines are either killed or attenuated. In order to ensure specificity, (1) the organisms employed for vaccine preparation must be from fresh cultures containing the immunogenic antigen and (2) this antigen must not be destroyed by heat or chemicals, frequently used in rendering the vaccine safe, or lost by prolonged cultivation during the process of attenuation.

The antigens of the genus *Salmonella* have been widely studied. In general, they consist of the lipopolysaccharide, somatic O antigens and the proteinaceous, flagellar H antigens. The more labile H antigens are readily destroyed by chemical or physical means and therefore it is simple to isolate the resistant O antigens. H antigens are not readily prepared in pure form, and in practice it is common to label preparations bearing flagella as H antigens, keeping in mind that the O antigens are present and intact though sometimes masked.

In the following experiment, *Salmonella* vaccines will be made, incorporating the above principles in their production. Similar procedures are used in the preparation of other bacterial vaccines.

PROCEDURE—H Antigens

1. Inoculate each of two vaccine bottles containing trypticase soy agar with a 1-ml portion of a broth culture of the assigned species of *Salmonella*. Make sure that all of the agar surface is covered with inoculum. Incubate the bottles, agar surface up, at 37°C for 24 hr.

2. Remove growth from one of the bottles with a 1-ml portion of formal-saline. Place the suspended growth in a large, sterile screw-cap tube.

3. Adjust the suspension by adding formal-saline so that the turbidity is between No. 3 and No. 4 of a McFarland's nephelometer tube (1 x 10⁹ organisms/ml).

4. Store at room temperature for 48 hr.

5. Test for sterility after 48 hr by aseptically transferring 1 drop of vaccine to 10 ml thioglycollate broth. Incubate for one week at 37°C.

PROCEDURE—O Antigens

1. Remove the contents of the second bottle with a 1-ml portion of absolute alcohol, and place it in a sterile screw-cap tube.

2. Heat the tube in a water bath at 60°C for 1 hr.

3. Centrifuge and discard the supernate.

4. Standardize to 1×10^9 organisms/ml, and check for sterility as in the section on the preparation of H antigens.

2. Viral Vaccines

Viruses, being obligate intracellular parasites, require living cells as substrate for their growth. Therefore, any active immunizing agent must first be prepared as the live infectious material in some natural or experimental host. A popular experimental animal for propagation of many viruses in relatively pure form is the embryonated chicken egg. Cell cultures of other animal tissues also serve as excellent substrates for the preparation of virus fluids of even greater purity.

The types of virus preparations that can be used for active immunization are basically the same as for bacterial vaccines. They are: (1) live attenuated, such as the smallpox, yellow fever, and oral poliomyelitis vaccines; (2) chemically inactivated, exemplified by the Salk type polio and egg embryo-produced influenza vaccines, both inactivated by formaldehyde; and (3) heat and ultraviolet irradiation inactivated. Formaldehyde is by far the most widely used killing agent. When used properly, it does not destroy the important antigenic component.

In the following experiment, influenza type A (Asian strain) will be propagated in the allantoic cavity of 11-day-old embryonated eggs and a vaccine prepared by inactivating the virus with formaldehyde.

PROCEDURE

1. Obtain two 11-day-old embryonated eggs.

2. Inoculate each egg with 0.2 ml virus suspension via the allantoic cavity. (The method of inoculation will be demonstrated.)

3. After inoculating and resealing the eggs, incubate without turning at 35°C for 48 to 96 hr. Discard any embryos that die within 24 hr.

4. After the embryos are dead, remove the eggs to a refrigerator for 1 to 2 hr.

5. Aseptically aspirate the allantoic fluid from each egg, and place the fluid in sterile centrifuge tubes. (This technique will be demonstrated.) Clarify by centrifugation.

6. Check supernatant for sterility by inoculating 10 ml thioglycollate broth with 1 ml fluid and incubating for 1 week at 37°C.

7. Remove a 3-ml aliquot from each sample and store it in the freezer for later estimation of virus content by the hemagglutination procedure (EXERCISE 8).

8. To the remaining portion of fluid in each vial, add sufficient formaldehyde to effect a final concentration of 0.4%. Incubate at 37°C for at least 1 hr and then in the refrigerator for 1 week. This preparation may be stored indefinitely at 4 to 6°C.

3. Erythrocyte Antigens

Erythrocyte suspensions are frequently used as immunizing agents in preparing such reagents as blood typing sera and hemolytic sensitizer for complement fixation tests. Only freshly drawn, uncontaminated whole blood should be used for this preparation.

PROCEDURE

1. Aseptically add 10 ml freshly citrated whole blood to a sterile 12-ml centrifuge tube.

2. Centrifuge at 2000 x g for 5 min.

3. Remove supernatant plasma.

4. Wash cells by adding sterile physiological saline to the original volume. Resuspend cells by gently shaking or stirring the tube.

5. Centrifuge as above and remove supernate. Repeat until three washings have been made.

6. Resuspend cells in sterile physiological saline to make a 10% suspension.

7. Transfer the suspension to a sterile stoppered container and store in the refrigerator. Disregard subsequent lysis if used within 3 to 4 weeks.

4. Protein Solutions

Protein solutions such as ovalbumin, serum, and plasma are readily prepared for immunization procedures to produce antisera. When mixed with the soluble antigen, this antiserum produces a precipitate. If a crystalline material is to be used for immunization, a 1% solution in saline is generally adequate. This must be sterilized by filtration before administration.

PROCEDURE

1. Aseptically place the desired volume of serum or plasma in a sterile centrifuge tube.

2. Centrifuge at 2000 x g until the supernate is clear of cellular debris.

3. Carefully transfer supernate to a sterile stoppered container.

4. Add enough 1/1000 aqueous Merthiolate (Eli Lilly and Co., Indianapolis, IN) to effect a final concentration of 1/10,000.

5. Adjuvants

Adjuvants are frequently used in immunizations to enhance the stimulation of antibody production. Adjuvants are thought to act by making the antigen either more particulate or more insoluble, thus holding the antigen in a depot and releasing it slowly over a long period of time. These substances may serve also to stimulate the proliferation of B-cell precursors in lymph nodes, spleen, and liver.

One of the most common adjuvants in use is that of Freund, which is a mixture of mineral oil and antigen that is emulsified in lanolin and to which killed tubercle bacilli have been added. The latter addition greatly increases the efficiency of the adjuvant by stimulating the proliferation of macrophages. Since hypersensitivity to the tuberculoprotein is produced in animals receiving the complete form of this adjuvant, repeated injections are made using antigen mixed with the incomplete form (without tubercle bacilli). Another disadvantage of this method is the production of sterile abscesses at the site of injection of the adjuvant. This property has made Freund's adjuvant unsuitable for human use.

Alum precipitation is another commonly used adjuvant. This procedure usually involves precipitating the protein antigen with aluminum potassium sulfate, which not only concentrates the antigen but also promotes phagocytosis.

PROCEDURE

A.   FREUND'S ADJUVANT

1.   Place 2 ml of Freund's complete adjuvant (Difco) into a 13-x-100-mm test tube. Add a small quantity of antigen to the adjuvant, and emulsify with a 5-ml syringe and a 20-gauge needle.

2.   Continue adding small amounts of antigen and emulsifying the mixture until a total of 2 ml of antigen has been added. The emulsion must be water-in-oil. The emulsion is satisfactory if a drop placed on a water surface does not spread.

3.   Administration varies with the animal. For rabbits, 2 ml of this preparation injected intramuscularly in each hind leg or subcutaneously in each of two sites at the back of the neck is adequate. Animals begin to respond after 3 to 4 weeks. If subsequent injections are necessary, emulsify the antigen in Freund's incomplete antigen.

B.   ALUM PRECIPITATION

The following method has been developed primarily for use with serum protein antigens.

1.   Dilute 5 ml serum with 16 ml distilled water.

2.   Add 18 ml 10% aluminum potassium sulfate and with constant stirring adjust the pH to 6.5 with 5 N NaOH.

3.   Centrifuge the precipitate and wash twice in saline. Add enough saline to bring the final volume up to 20 ml.

4.   A 5-ml intramuscular injection into each hind leg of a rabbit should produce a high precipitin titer in 2 to 3 weeks.

6.   Immunization Schedules

Many of the antisera used in these exercises can easily be prepared by students. Although individual immunization procedures vary, the following schedules have generally been adequate:

1.   BACTERIAL SUSPENSIONS (1×10^9 organisms/ml)

Day 1	0.1	ml I.V.
Day 3	0.25	ml I.V.
Day 5	0.5	ml I.V.
Day 8	1.0	ml I.V.
Day 10	1.0	ml I.V.
Day 12	1.0	ml I.V.
Day 15	1.0	ml I.V.
Day 17	1.0	ml I.V.
Day 19	1.0	ml I.V.

One week after the last injection, give the animal a trial bleeding and check the serum titer. If a satisfactory titer is obtained, the animal's blood may be collected; otherwise inject 1 ml antigen and rebleed after 5 to 7 days.

2. VIRAL VACCINES

Day 1	0.5 ml I.V.
Day 3	0.5 ml I.V.
Day 5	1.0 ml I.V.
Day 8	1.0 ml I.V.
Day 15	1.0 ml I.V.
Day 22	1.0 ml I.V.

One week after the last injection, make a trial bleeding and examine as before. If the titer is sufficient, the animal's blood may be collected.

3. ERYTHROCYTE SUSPENSIONS (10%)

Day 1	1.0 ml I.V.
Day 2	1.0 ml I.V.
Day 3	1.0 ml I.V.
Day 5	1.0 ml I.V.
Day 7	1.0 ml I.V.
Day 10	1.0 ml I.V.

Seven to ten days after the last injection, the animal may be trial bled as above. If the titer is insufficient, rebleed the following week.

4. PROTEIN SOLUTIONS (1%)

Day 1	0.1 ml I.V.
Day 3	0.5 ml I.V.
Day 5	1.0 ml I.V.
Day 8	1.0 ml I.V.
Day 10	1.0 ml I.V. CAUTION
Day 12	1.0 ml I.V. CAUTION
Day 15	1.0 ml I.V. CAUTION
Day 17	1.0 ml I.V. CAUTION
Day 19	1.0 ml I.V. CAUTION

The animal may be given a trial bleeding after either of the last two injections.

CAUTION: After the first week, the antigen should be either given intraperitoneally or combined with an antihistamine to reduce the possibility of anaphylactic shock.

Immunization Schedule

Antigen	Date	Amount Injected	Mode	Remarks

Final titer _____

Each student will be assigned an animal and an antiserum to prepare. Use the above table to record the data concerning each injection. Report any signs of ill health of the animal to the instructor. After the final titration, record the results in the table.

All antisera used in these experiments with the exception of the commercial typing sera will be made by students in the class. The sera that you make will be used in experiments by students taking the course in the future. Similarly, students preceding you prepared the sera that you will be using. By careful inventory and planning, the instructor should be able to make antiserum assignments that will supply future needs.

7. Animal Techniques

The care and maintenance of animals is subject to a great many governmental regulations and controls.[1] Also, many people misinterpret what they see and hear about animals being used for scientific purposes. To avoid restrictive legislation, scientists must pay strict attention to animal handling and treatment. Aside from restrictive legislation, we have a responsibility to spare animals any needless pain and to treat them in a humane manner. The following simple technique will be demonstrated:

Rabbits: Rabbits are large enough and have sufficient muscular strength that they can inflict severe injury on the operator or themselves. Great care must be taken in picking rabbits up and carrying them. Place your hand over the pelvic girdle and grab a generous amount of the loose skin, not just the superficial fur, and firmly turn the rabbit, rear end toward you. If the animal is in a cage, its natural tendency is to grab onto the mesh floor. To avoid this, tilt your hand grasping the rabbit 90° and pull it straight out. Immediately place the head and forequarters under your opposite arm and gently but firmly pin the rabbit

[1] "Guide for the Care and Use of Laboratory Animals," NIH Publication No. 80-23. USPHS, 1978.

to your side while continuing your grasp of the skin over the hindquarters. This will prevent the animal from arching its back too quickly and injuring itself. If the animal is picked up over the middle of its vertebral column, it will flex its powerful rear legs and back muscles, liberally scratching anything in the way, but worse, breaking its own back. This is an inexcusable injury, and the rabbit will have to be killed rather than be allowed to live paralyzed.

All animals should be marked in some permanent manner. Most methods involve tagging the ear. Care should be taken to avoid puncturing the major blood vessels or placing any tag in such a position that it obscures the lateral ear veins. If a small incision or hole must be made to accommodate a tag, the operation must be performed quickly and firmly as gentleness at this point will only cause needless pain to the animal.

When performing any injection or treatment, have an assistant properly restrain the animal or place it in a device designed for the purpose. If an assistant is employed, he or she should press the hindquarters flat against the table and, while standing parallel to the animal, place one arm on the far side of it. The assistant should firmly squeeze the animal, using the elbow at the hindquarters and the hand at the shoulders. The assistant should use both hands to form a collar around the animal's neck and shoulders, holding the thumbs at the top of the head where it is simple to use them to deflect one of the rabbit's ears toward the operator for injection purposes.

Other means of temporary restraint will be demonstrated for making intramuscular and intraperitoneal injections, as well as means of restraint for extended operations.

The intravenous injection is one of the most common methods of administering antigen to rabbits because of the accessibility of large veins in this species. The lateral ear vein can accommodate needles up to 18 gauge in size, although the smaller 27- to 22-gauge needles are usually preferred. After placing the animal in restraint, dilate the lateral ear vein by blocking off venous backflow and gently irritating the area. Wetting the ear down with alcohol does not effectively kill bacteria, but it does improve visibility of the vein. Firmly hold the ear with one hand and insert the needle, bevel side up, into the vein, keeping the needle as parallel as possible to the plane of the vein. Gently push on the syringe plunger. If any resistance is felt, the needle is not in the vein. When properly inserted, the plunger will meet no resistance, and the vein can be observed to clear upon injection of the fluid.

The following methods of injection, all useful in immunization procedures, will be demonstrated: intradermal, foot pad, subcutaneous, intramuscular, and intraperitoneal.

Guinea pigs: Guinea pigs are usually immunized by methods other than intravenous injection. Intradermal injection in this animal is quite common and is accomplished by use of a 27-gauge needle. After shaving a small area of skin on the side of the guinea pig, wet down the remaining guard hairs with alcohol. The injection is made by firmly placing the bevel of the needle just under and within the most superficial layer of the skin. Upon injecting from 0.03 to 0.1 ml into the skin, you should note the formation of a distinct bleb or blister. If not, you have injected subcutaneously and too deeply.

Your instructor will demonstrate the handling, restraint, and bleeding of other common laboratory animals (e.g., mice, chickens, and hamsters), emphasizing safety and humane treatment.

Exercise 3

INNATE IMMUNITY

Immunity can be broadly classified into two categories—innate and acquired. Classical acquired immunity involves the presence of antibody or specific lymphocytes and is the kind with which most of this manual is concerned. However, animals possess an innate or constitutional immunity that is even more important. This type of immunity has nothing to do with specific immune effectors, is genetically inherited, and is constant for all members of a species. It cannot be passively transferred or otherwise acquired. Some of the more important aspects of this facet of total immunity will be considered here.

1. Bactericidal Power of Normal Serum

Fresh normal serum contains substances capable of killing microorganisms. This ability varies with the species and type of microorganism. To be sure, some of this activity may be due to spontaneously acquired antibodies, but other humoral factors are also involved. For instance, unheated fresh serum contains a series of proteins known as complement, some of which under certain conditions play a role in the elimination or destruction of foreign particles. Some of these proteins can be inactivated if the serum is preheated at 56°C for 30 min (these will be studied in more detail later). Lactoferrin, C-reactive protein, and antivasin are other examples of known humoral factors that contribute to innate immunity. This experiment demonstrates the combined effects of these substances on some common bacteria.

PROCEDURE

1. Twenty-four-hour broth cultures (Trypticase soy or brain-heart infusion broths) of *Salmonella paratyphi* and *Staphylococcus aureus* will be used as the indicator organisms. The instructor will assign one of the cultures to each pair of students.

2. Prepare five dilutions of each organism in sterile saline as follows:

    a. 0.1 ml culture   into 9.9 ml sterile saline—1/100
    b. 0.1 ml 1/100   into 9.9 ml sterile saline—1/10,000
    c. 1.0 ml 1/10,000   into 9.9 ml sterile saline—1/100,000
    d. 1.0 ml 1/100,000 into 9.9 ml sterile saline—1/1,000,000
    e. 1.0 ml 1/1 million into 9.9 ml sterile saline—1/10,000,000

    CAUTION: Do not pipette pathogens by mouth.

3. Using aseptic technique, set up three tubes for each of the three highest dilutions as follows:

    a. Normal unheated serum   0.5 ml
        Culture dilution   0.5 ml

    b. Normal heated serum (56°C/30 min)   0.5 ml
        Culture dilution   0.5 ml

c. Sterile saline   0.5 ml
     Culture dilution   0.5 ml

4. Mix the contents of all tubes (nine per organism) well and incubate in a 37°C water bath for 1 hr.

5. After incubation, place the contents of each tube into a sterile Petri dish, labeled accordingly.

6. Pour 10 ml melted (45°C) Trypticase soy or brain-heart infusion agar into each plate and gently agitate so as to effect an even distribution of organisms in the medium.

7. After the agar has hardened, incubate all plates at 37°C for 36 to 48 hr.

8. After incubation, carefully make plate counts of all countable plates and record the results.

9. Make comparisons and explain the results.

Organism	Number of Viable Organisms Remaining	
	Heated Serum	*Unheated Serum*

2. Clearance of Blood by the Reticuloendothelial System

Innate immunity is also largely influenced by cellular factors in the animal body. The most important of these is phagocytosis or the engulfment of foreign particles by the leukocytes and other cells of the reticulo-endothelial system. The cellular aspects of immunity are intimately associated with the antibody aspects and will be considered in this regard in more detail in EXERCISES 5 and 19.

Apart from their association with antibodies, the cells and tissues of the reticuloendothelial system constitute a vast and widely disseminated apparatus that effectively filters foreign particles from the circulating blood as this blood passes through organs containing phagocytes. In this experiment, living bacteria will be used as an indicator to determine where in the body such particles are removed from the circulation.

PROCEDURE

This experiment will be conducted by the class. The instructor will assign to students or groups of students certain portions of this experiment. At the conclusion, the results will be pooled in the composite table following the instructions.

1. Determine the number of bacteria present in the blood of a rabbit immediately after intravenous injection of 100 million bacteria of *Escherichia coli*.

   a. Prepare 1/1000, 1/10,000, and 1/100,000 dilutions of the blood sample.

   b. Prepare pour plates using 1 ml of the above dilutions.

2. Determine the number of bacteria present in the blood of a rabbit 30 min after injection.

   a. Prepare 1/10, 1/100, and 1/1000 dilutions of the blood sample.

   b. Prepare pour plates using 1 ml of the above dilutions.

3. Determine the number of bacteria present in the blood of the rabbit 60 min after injection.

   a. Prepare 1/10 and 1/100 dilutions of the blood sample.

   b. Prepare pour plates using 1 ml of the above dilutions and 1 ml whole blood.

4. Determine the number of bacteria present in the liver, lungs, spleen, and heart of the rabbit 60 min after the injection.

   a. Place 1 g of each organ in a sterile mortar on a Waring blender and add 100 ml sterile saline. Make a suspension of the organ.

   b. Prepare 1/100, 1/1000, and 1/10,000 dilutions of each organ suspension.

   c. Prepare pour plates using 1 ml of the above dilutions.

Let all plates harden and then incubate at 37°C for 48 hr. After incubation, make plate counts and record the data in the following table. Explain the results.

Sample	Time	Organisms/ml
Blood	Immediately	
Blood	30 min	
Blood	60 min	
Heart	60 min	
Liver	60 min	
Lungs	60 min	
Spleen	60 min	

3. Phagocytosis

The cellular line of defense is closely linked with that of the humoral line. Phagocytosis, or the engulfment of foreign particles by certain cells of the reticuloendothelial system, is markedly enhanced by the presence of certain antibodies. Proteins that render antigens susceptible to phagocytosis are termed opsonins. Such antibodies can be shown to increase during immunization and are dependent on the mediation of complement in their action.

In many ways, phagocytosis is the most important line of defense. Even with adequate amounts of antibodies and complement being present, the animal cannot survive with a defect in the phagocytic cells.

Several phagocytic defect syndromes are known in humans. The results of the previous experiment illustrate the effectiveness of phagocytic cells that line the channels and sinusoids of organs bearing lymphoid tissue. The following two experiments illustrate the morphology of peripherally circulating cells.

A. LEUKOCYTE DIFFERENTIAL COUNTS

In the circulating blood, a variety of leukocytes may be found. Actually, only certain kinds of these are phagocytic. These cells are classified largely by their morphology and their reactions when stained by Wright's stain. An increase or a decrease in the percentage of the leukocyte types may indicate certain pathological processes. By counting 100 representative leukocytes and recording the incidence of the specific kinds, such differential counts are easily ascertained. This experiment assumes that the student is familiar with the nomenclature and morphology of the various leukocytes (see FIGURE 3.1).

FIGURE 3.1

		Nucleus		Cytoplasm	
		Shape	*Chromatin*	*Ground Substance*	*Granules*
Neutrophil (65%) 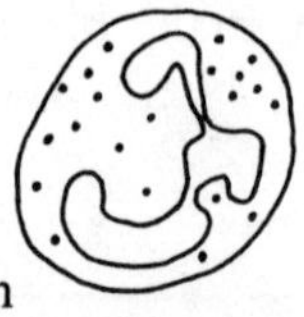 size: 9-12 μm		2-5 lobed united by thin filaments or broad bands	Fish-scale appearance; dark blue-deep purple	Pale lilac acidophilic	Neutral, deeper lilac; equal sized, fine
Eosinophiles (4%-5%) 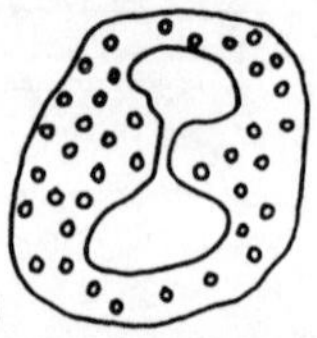 size: 9-12 μm		Usually 2 lobed	Blue-red to blue	Pale lilac acidophilic	Acid reaction; deep pink; equal sized, large, coarse refractive
Basophiles (less than 1%) 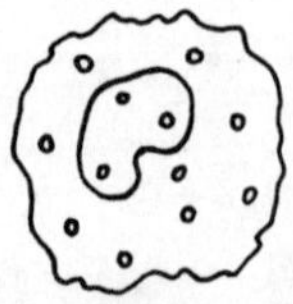 size: 9-12 μm		Rosette shaped or slightly polymorph	Gives hazy appearance; pale blue	More pinkish	Basic reaction; round, coarse, equal sized, few in number; deep bluish-purple
Monocytes (2%-4%) 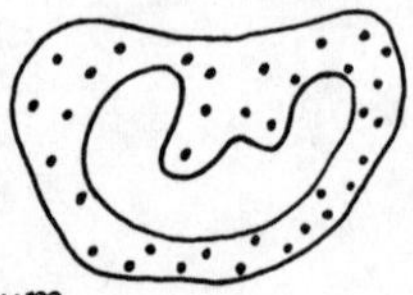 size: 14-18 μm		Bean shaped	Loosely meshed interlacing strands; pale blue	Basophilic gray-blue	Muddy blue, non-specific granules; "ground glass" appearance
Lymphocytes (25%) 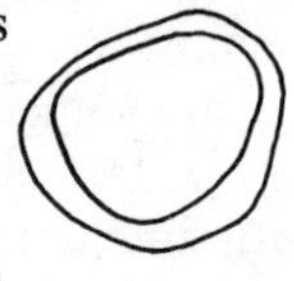 size: 7-13 μm		Round or oval, shallow or deeply indented	Demarcation not distinct, very coarse; dark blue	Slight amount clear blue light area around nucleus	May contain granules which are nonspecific; azure

PROCEDURE

1. Place a small drop (0.5 ml) of fresh blood on one end of a clean microscope slide.

2. Quickly make a smear of this drop by drawing out a film with the edge of another slide.

3. After the film has dried, stain with Wright's stain.

4. Examine the stained smears microscopically with the oil-immersion objective. Count 100 leukocytes from representative areas of the slide and record the incidence of each of the following types:

Lymphocytes	_____
Monocytes	_____
Neutrophils	_____
Eosinophils	_____
Basophils	_____
Total	100

B. DEMONSTRATION *IN VIVO*

PROCEDURE

1. Inject a mouse intraperitoneally with 0.25 ml of a suspension of *Staphylococcus aureus*.

2. Sacrifice the mouse with chloroform 30 to 45 min after the injection.

3. Aseptically autopsy the mouse, and carefully remove the liver.

4. Make impression smears of the peritoneal exudate and from cut surfaces of the liver.

5. After the smears dry, stain them with Wright's stain.

6. Observe the phagocytes microscopically for the presence of intracellular cocci, using the oil-immersion objective.

4. Phagocytic Dysfunction

Normal polymorphonuclear neutrophils (PMNs) rapidly kill most engulfed bacteria by low pH, enzymes, and hydrogen peroxide. Engulfed particles are enclosed within phagosomes, which converge with lysosomes. These latter structures disgorge into the phagosome enzymes (e.g., hydrolases, myeloperoxidase, and cationic proteins), which are mostly digestive enzymes. The most important part of the killing mechanism is the mediation of H_2O_2 produced through the hexose monophosphate shunt of normal glucose metabolism.

Diphosphopyridine nucleotide (NADH)-oxidase is the key enzyme for producing peroxide, and in this experiment, hydrocortisone-21-succinate, a potent inhibitor of this enzyme, is used to make peroxide-deficient neutrophils. Possibly, the beneficial, anti-inflammatory effects of chemotherapy with steroids are due to a similar mechanism. The leukocytes rendered nonfunctional by this method resemble those naturally found in chronic granulomatous disease, an immunodeficient syndrome characterized by failure of the patient's leukocytes to kill bacteria because of deficient peroxide production.

PROCEDURE

Use aseptic technique and sterile glassware throughout.

1. Prepare ahead of time the following:

    a. An 18-hr Trypticase soy broth (Difco) culture of *Staphylococcus aureus* that has been washed twice in sterile saline, resuspended in 10 ml saline, and 0.1 ml of this diluted 1/100.

    b. A filter sterilized sedimentation gradient solution composed of 6% dextran (M.W. 100,000-200,000) containing 50 units of heparin/ml.

2. Draw no more than 10 ml human blood into a sterile, heparinized syringe.

3. Layer with 1 ml sedimentation solution and incubate for 1 hr at R°. Withdraw the supernate.

4. Centrifuge the supernate at 800 g for 8 min. This will sediment most, but not all, of the white cells. Decant supernate and save.

5. Resuspend cells in heparinized saline and proceed to step 7.

6. Further clarify plasma from step 4 for use in steps 9 and 10.

7. Wash twice in sterile heparinized saline (25 units/100 ml) at 400 g for 6 min each or until the supernates are clear.

8. Resuspend the button in exactly 7.2 ml of Hanks balanced salt solution.

9. Divide the cell suspension evenly between two sterile tubes. To one tube add 0.4 ml plasma from step 5. This is the control.

10. To the other tube add 0.4 ml plasma from step 5 in which you have dissolved 4 mg hydrocortisone-21-succinate (Sigma). This will be the inhibition test.

11. To each tube add 0.2 ml 1/100 *S. aureus* suspension from step 1a.

12. Mix well and incubate for 60 min at 37°C with frequent shaking.

13. Remove 1-ml samples immediately, at 30 min and at 60 min (work in groups), and prepare 1/10, 1/100, and 1/1000 dilutions from these samples.

14. Plate 1-ml samples from each dilution, and incubate at 37°C for 24 to 48 hr.

15. Make plate counts, and compare the killing curves between the test and the cortisone-treated cells. Confirmation that the treated cells have actually engulfed the bacteria may be made by Wright's staining a drop of the test sample.

5. Nitroblue Tetrazolium (NBT) Reduction Assay

When neutrophiles phagocytize particles, a burst in oxidative metabolism results in the generation of oxygen radicals that have microbiocidal activity. One of the simplest and most direct methods of detecting this metabolic change is the NBT reduction assay, wherein the yellowish NBT is reduced to an insoluble, purplish precipitate in the phagolysosomes. The test is useful in the detection of defects in the oxidative metabolism of neutrophiles, such as that seen in individuals with chronic granulomatous disease.

PROCEDURE

1. Draw 1 ml human blood into a heparinized syringe.

2. Place 0.1 ml into each of two small tubes or wells of concave microscope slides.

3. If cortisone-treated PMNs have been prepared for EXPERIMENT 4 above, place 0.1 ml into two other tubes.

4. Add 0.1 ml freshly prepared 0.2% NBT solution to each sample.

5. Add 0.05 ml bacterial suspension (e.g., the suspension prepared in step 1a in EXPERIMENT 4 above) to one of the tubes in each pair.

6. Incubate at 37°C for 15 to 30 min in a humidity chamber.

7. After the incubation, gently suspend with a capillary pipette and prepare a blood smear from each sample.

8. Stain the slides with Wright's stain and examine under an oil-immersion objective.

9. Positive cells will contain large, purplish-blue granules (formazan) with refractile edges. In normal individuals, 5% to 10% of unstimulated PMNs will possess these granules, but this value should increase to nearly 50% in the presence of a phagocytic stimulus.

Treatment	Total Number of Cells	NBT Positive Cells	Percent NBT Positive
Bacteria Present			
Bacteria Absent			

6. Superoxide Anion Production

The microbiocidal activity of phagocytic cells (monocytes, macrophages, and neutrophils) is largely due to the generation of oxygen metabolites and free radicals such as hydrogen peroxide, hydroxyl radicals, and superoxide anion. Measurement of the production of these compounds can be used as an indirect measure of the ability of these cells to kill microbes. In this experiment, the generation of the superoxide anion will be monitored based upon the reduction of cytochrome C by this oxygen-free radical. The phagocytic cells (neutrophils, in this case) will be stimulated to produce superoxide anion by the addition of opsonized zymosan particles. The production of the oxygen radical will be monitored over time.

PROCEDURE

NOTE: Because of the large number of cells required, it is recommended that this be done as a group or class experiment.

1. Draw 30 ml blood into a syringe containing 1000 units heparin.

2. Mix the blood with 10 ml 6% sedimentation media (6% dextran, 100,000 to 200,000 M.W., in saline). This can be done directly in the syringe or in a tall, narrow cylinder.

3. Incubate at R° for 45 to 60 min, and recover the opalescent supernate. This will contain the leukocytes.

4. Wash the leukocyte suspension three times with Hanks balanced salt solution (HBSS) by centrifuging at 1000 x g for 5 min and resuspending the cells in HBSS.

5. After the last wash, resuspend the cells in 5 ml HBSS.

6. Set up the assay according to the following protocol. Tubes should be incubated in a shaking 37°C-water bath or frequently mixed by hand.

Tube Number	HBSS	Cytochrome C	Zymosan	Cells
1	8 ml	1 ml	1 ml	—
2	8 ml	1 ml	—	1 ml
3	7 ml	1 ml	1 ml	1 ml

7. Mix the reactants, and immediately remove a 2-ml sample from each tube. This is the time 0 sample. Separate the supernate from the cells by either filtering through a 0.45 μ filter or by centrifugation at 10,000 rpm for 1 min.

8. Remove 2-ml samples from each tube after 5, 15, and 30 min of incubation, and process as above.

9. Record the absorbance at 550 nm of the supernate samples, and plot the absorbance versus time.

Exercise 4

IMMUNOGLOBULINS

Immunoglobulins are the molecules of immunity, the humoral antibodies. Originally, antibodies were studied according to their solubility and electrophoretic mobility. Thus, since antibodies were electrophoretically slow-moving proteins, insoluble in distilled water, but soluble in weak electrolytes, they were called beta and gamma globulins. With improved methods of separation (e.g., more sophisticated electrophoresis techniques, ultracentrifugation, and ion-exchange chromatography), different systems of nomenclature were proposed and soon the whole terminology was in a mess. Finally, the early work on the enzymatic cleavage of antibody molecules resulted in further differences in the nomenclature of reaction products, which led to the development of a unified system of immunoglobulin nomenclature.

All antibody molecules or their basic units are composed of two pairs of chains, one pair being considerably larger than the other, leading to the designations, heavy and light chains (FIGURE 4.1).

FIGURE 4.1. Antibody Molecular Chains

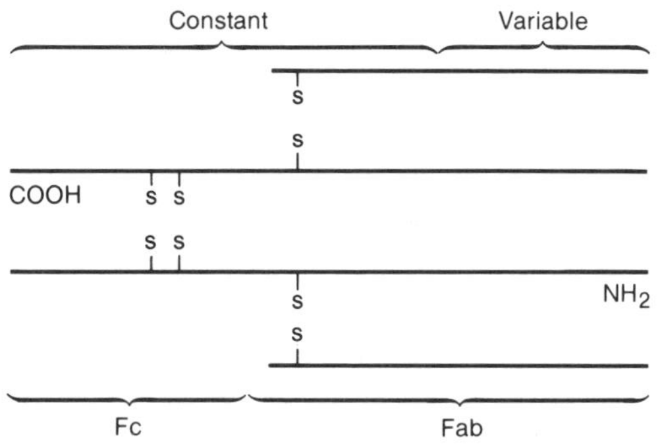

When an antibody molecule is hydrolyzed with papain, it breaks into three pieces, two separate but identical Fab fragments that contain one antigen-binding site each and one heavier Fc fragment, which has different functions depending on the nature of the heavy chain. Note that the antigen-binding ends of the chains are amino terminal portions and that the two chains in each Fab fragment are still linked together with disulfide linkages. The Fc fragment is composed of only heavy chain portions similarly linked, and its activity is through the carboxy terminal portion of the chains.

When an antibody molecule is digested with pepsin, only the carboxy terminal ends of the heavy chains are hydrolyzed distal to the disulfide linkage, leaving a single fragment with two antigen combining sites, the $F(ab')_2$.

All light chains are basically of two types, lambda (λ) and kappa (κ). Although each individual possesses a certain proportion of immunoglobulins with κ light chains (60%) and another proportion of λ chains (30%), both light chains in a single molecule are of the same type.

Currently five types of heavy chains are recognized, and each type determines the immunoglobulin class of that molecule. The heavy chains differ biochemically, serologically, and biologically. A table summarizing the different classes of heavy chains appears below:

Ig Class	*Heavy Chain*	*Characteristics*
IgG	γ	Mature antibody Fix complement Cross placenta Higher avidity
IgA	α	Secretory antibody
IgM	μ	Fix complement Initial antibody Higher specificity
IgD	δ	Maturational functions
IgE	ϵ	Fixes to mast cells

These immunoglobulins have different immunologic functions and serologic properties that are influenced by the nature of the pair of heavy chains in their structures.

A division can be made in either the heavy or light chain on amino acid sequencing. The first 110 amino acids on the amino terminal portion of each chain house the antigen reacting portion. This is called the variable region of the chain because antibodies of different specificity can be shown to have different types and sequences of amino acids in this portion. The amino acid types and sequences in the rest of the chains are remarkably constant from molecule to molecule, even across immunoglobulin classes and species lines.

The individual serologic properties of the different immunoglobulins will be pointed out in the various exercises of this manual. The following experiments demonstrate some of the basic chemical and biological properties of immunoglobulins.

1. Ultracentrifugation of Macroglobulins

The purpose of this experiment is to examine properties of the IgM class of immunoglobulins. This class has a molecular weight of about 1 million and thus sediments faster in the ultracentrifuge than the other immunoglobulins. It does not pass the placenta, but may be synthesized *in utero*. IgM is characteristic of the primary response and is the most efficient antibody in causing agglutination. Basically, it is a pentamer composed of five separate units held together covalently by additional peptides.

These linkages are easily broken by mild reduction with mercaptoethanol, causing the molecule to lose its effectiveness as an agglutinating agent. IgG is unaffected by such treatment because strong noncovalent forces hold the chains intact even after the interchain disulfide bonds have been reduced. Thus, mercaptoethanol affords a simple and convenient way to distinguish these two classes.

PROCEDURE

1. For this experiment, use a serum in which a known, easily detectable macroglobulin is present (e.g., rheumatoid factor, cold agglutinin, or infectious mononucleosis agglutinin). The appropriate titer of the unfractionated serum should also be known.

2. This experiment requires a preparatory ultracentrifuge with a swinging bucket rotor and cellulose nitrate tubes. The use of the ultracentrifuge will be demonstrated.

3. Into the bottom of each tube, carefully deposit 1.5 ml 37% sucrose solution in PBS.

4. Next, carefully layer an equal amount of 25% sucrose solution in PBS over the previous solution. Do not mix.

5. Finally, layer in similar fashion 1.5 ml 10% sucrose solution in PBS. Allow these tubes to sit undisturbed for 24 hr at 4°C.

6. Gently mix 0.5 ml 1/2 dilution of the serum sample into the top layer.

7. Insert the tubes in the rotor, place the rotor in the centrifuge, and slowly bring the rotor to 35,000 rpm over a 5-min period. Centrifuge at this speed for 18 hr.

8. Stop the centrifuge with the brake off. When the rotor has come to a complete stop, remove the tubes carefully from the rotor.

9. Puncture the bottom of each tube with a 26-gauge needle and collect the first six drops. Label this fraction F1.

10. Discard the next 8 drops, F2, from each tube, but collect the next 20 drops and label this portion F3.

11. Retitrate the F1 and F3 fractions against the appropriate antigen.

12. From the F1 and F3 fractions of a separate tube, mix a 0.2-ml portion of each with an equal volume of 0.2 M solution of mercaptoethanol, a substance known to degrade macroglobulins.

13. Allow the mixtures to stand for 24 hr at room temperature and retitrate. Consider the dilutions that have been made when assaying the results of the titers.

2. Immunoglobulin Quantitation

Immunoglobulins are easily quantitated by means of simple precipitation reactions in gels. Because the heavy chains are in themselves antigenically distinct, highly specific antisera may be prepared against each chain. A known amount of heavy chain-specific antiserum is incorporated into an agar solution which in turn is poured into a microscope slide. Upon hardening, the agar is punched with small holes. If a hole is charged with serum containing the immunoglobulin in question, a halo of serologic precipitation will form around the hole as the serum diffuses. The diameter of the halo is directly proportional to the concentration of the immunoglobulin.

PROCEDURE

1. For this experiment, obtain some commercially prepared immunodiffusion plates specific for one of the immunoglobulin classes.

2. Fill three of the wells with sera of known amounts of the desired immunoglobulin. Three concentrations should be selected to form a broad range. Carefully fill the wells even with the top, taking care not to allow any to run over. For best results, the wells should be filled to the same height using the capillary pipettes provided.

3. Into the other wells, introduce equal amounts of unknown sera. If available, use sera from an immunodeficient patient or a patient with a myeloma of the class in question.

4. Incubate the plates overnight at room temperature in a moist chamber.

5. Measure the diameter of precipitation around each well with either a special viewer designed for the purpose or a dissecting microscope fitted with an ocular micrometer.

6.   Using 2-cycle semilogarithmic paper (as shown in FIGURE 4.2), plot the squares of the diameters of the knowns on the arithmetic scale versus their respective concentrations on the logarithmic scale. A straight line should result.

7.   Obtain the concentrations of the unknowns from the graph.

FIGURE 4.2. Two-cycle Semilogarithmic Graph

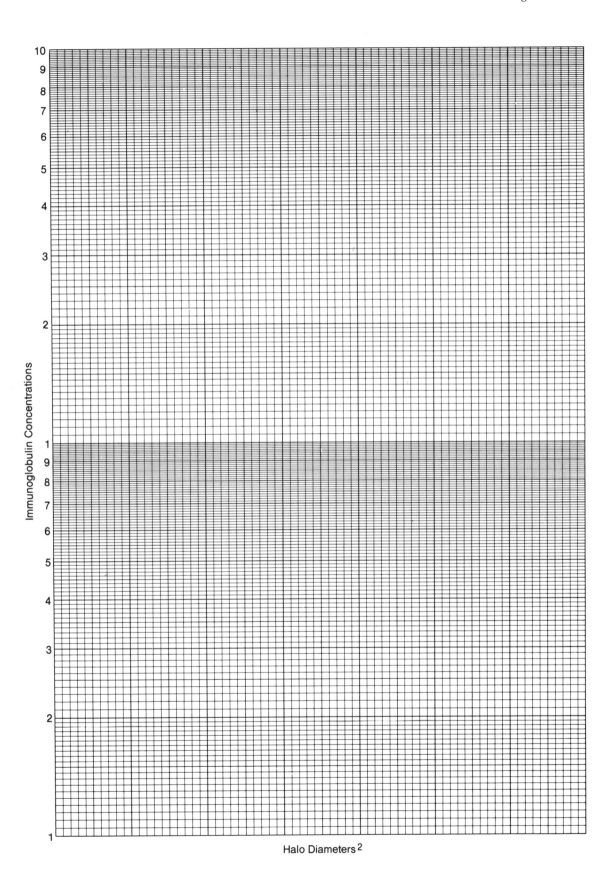

Immunoglobulin Concentrations

Halo Diameters ^{2}

Exercise 5

T-CELL AND B-CELL IMMUNITY

Perhaps the greatest change in our understanding of immunology during the last 20 years has been in the area of the cellular immune response. The concept of two distinct lymphocyte populations that operate in concert, yet have different effector mechanisms and appear to have separate evolutionary origins, forms the modern backbone of this understanding of the cellular basis for immunity.

The humoral arm of the immune system is known as the B-cell, bursal dependent or bone marrow dependent, system. The humoral mechanism is concentrated in all avian species in an outpocketing of gastrointestinal epithelium known as the Bursa of Fabricius. If this organ is removed soon after hatching, the chick will be deficient in germinal center development of lymph nodes, plasma cells, and immunoglobulins. Mammals do not have such a centrally-located, analogous organ. Rather, the fetal liver and spleen and adult bone marrow appear to be the sites of B-cell development in mammals. B-lymphocytes that arise from these origins populate the secondary lymphoid organs (e.g., lymph nodes, spleen, and Peyer's patches), and upon antigenic stimulation differentiate into immunoglobulin-producing plasma cells. B-cells are identified by the presence of immunoglobulins on their cell membrane surfaces. Immature B-cells express IgM or IgD molecules (or both), but appropriate stimulation can induce a class switch such that IgG, IgA, or IgE may be found. Identification of immunoglobulin molecules on the surface of lymphocytes allows for the recognition and quantitation of this type of lymphocyte in blood or lymphoid organs.

The other main arm of the immune system is referred to as the T-cell, or thymus dependent system. This component of the immune system is responsible for certain cell-mediated forms of immunity as well as certain immunoregulatory functions. Because T-cell development occurs in the thymus, thymectomy of neonatal animals deprives them of this type of immune function and leaves them vulnerable to secondary, intracellular infections. T-cells have been shown to play critical roles in the initiation, regulation, and expression of the immune response. At least three subpopulations of T-cells are known: helper cells, suppressor cells, and cytotoxic (or effector) cells. Helper and suppressor cells are involved in the induction and regulation of both humoral and cellular responses, while the cytotoxic cells are responsible for various defensive functions against specific targets.

In a humoral immune response, T- and B-cells act in concert to generate an efficient response to many kinds of antigens. For example, T-cells regulate the quantity and quality of the antibody response of B-cells. In addition, a third class of cells known collectively as macrophages plays an essential role in generating immune responses. These cells phagocytize, process, and present antigens to T-cells, which is the critical event in the initiation of immune response to many kinds of antigens. Moreover, they may become "activated" by lymphocyte products to become more effective phagocytic cells with enhanced microbiocidal activity. A macrophage has on its surface receptors for such molecules as the Fc portion of certain immunoglobulins. These receptors enable the cell to recognize and engulf antigen-antibody complexes more readily.

1. Enumeration of B- and T-Cells in Blood

Although B- and T-cells are morphologically identical, they can be differentiated on the basis of specific membrane-associated molecules. Taking advantage of the immunoglobulin expression on the cell membranes, one can use fluorescent-labeled antiglobulins to identify and enumerate B-cells. One would have to use an ultraviolet-illuminated microscope, however, to observe stained cells. An alternative method of identifying the B-cells is to use latex beads coated with antibodies to human immunoglobulins. These beads will stick to any cell bearing immunoglobulins and may be observed with a conventional microscope.

Human T-cells are easily identified on the basis of a membrane receptor that binds to sheep erythrocytes. Although the physiological significance of this receptor is not known, it affords a convenient method of identifying T-cells in mixtures by causing them to form "rosettes" when the erythrocytes adhere to their surfaces.

PROCEDURE

1. Draw 10 ml human blood into 1000 units heparin in a 20-ml syringe.

2. Add 10 ml PBS to the sample, and mix thoroughly. This may be done in the syringe or a large tube.

3. Place 4 ml sedimentation medium into each of four 17-x-100-mm test tubes.

4. Carefully layer 5 ml blood onto the surface of the sedimentation medium. Avoid mixing the blood and the separation medium.

5. Centrifuge at 400 x g for 30 min at room temperature. After centrifugation, the leukocytes will appear as a fluffy, white band at the plasma-medium interface, while the erythrocytes will be on the bottom of the tube below the medium.

6. Carefully remove as much as possible of the topmost layer of plasma with a capillary pipette, and recentrifuge thoroughly.

7. Remove the white cells, taking as little as possible of the separation medium from the lower layer.

8. Wash the white cells by suspending them in PBS, centrifuging for 6 min at 400 x g, and resuspending them in PBS. Repeat three times.

9. After the last wash, resuspend the cells in 0.5 ml PBS containing 0.05 ml autologous plasma (from step 5).

T-Cell Enumeration

a. Wash a suspension of sheep erythrocytes (SRBCs) three times and resuspend to a concentration of 4×10^7/ml (about 0.1 ml of packed cells in 5 ml phosphate buffered saline).

b. Mix together 0.1 ml of the lymphocyte-plasma mixture (from step 8) and 0.1 ml SRBCs.

c. Incubate at 37°C for 15 min, centrifuge at 200 x g for 1 hr, and then reincubate at 4°C for 1 hr with the supernate still on the pellet.

d. *Very* gently resuspend the cells by tilting the tube back and forth two or three times. Fill a hemocytometer with suspended cells and count 200 lymphocytes, keeping track of the proportion of rosettes or cells with more than three SRBCs adhering to them.

e. If the SRBC concentration is too high, it will be difficult to count the rosettes. Try using fewer SRBCs if this occurs. The optimal ratio should be 8:1, SRBCs to lymphocytes.

B-Cell Enumeration

$\pi^{\frac{1}{4}}$

a. Prepare a suspension of Immunobeads according to the manufacturer's directions.

b. Mix 0.1 ml lymphocyte suspension (from step 8) with 0.1 ml Immunobeads.

c. Incubate for 1 hr at 4°C.

d. Gently resuspend the suspension, and fill a hemocytometer as above. Count 200 lymphocytes, keeping track of the number with beads adhering to them.

Assay	*Total Number of Cells Counted*	*E Rosette or Immunobead Positive*	*Percent Positive*
T-Cells	200		
B-Cells	200	33 Immunobead positive	

2.   Demonstration of B-Cell Dependent Function

The hallmark of B-cell activation is the production of antibody molecules. A clever way to detect cells that produce specific antibody for erythrocytes is to use a plaque assay on spleen-cell suspensions from immunized animals. Spleen cells from mice immunized with SRBCs are mixed with the erythrocytes. In the presence of complement, antibody secreted by the cells is bound to erythrocytes and results in the appearance of a zone of lysis around those cells. Two methods of performing the assay are presented. The first is the more traditional method, which employs the use of an agar overlay in which the plaques form. The second is a modification that does not require agar and uses much smaller quantities of reagents.

PROCEDURE

1. Strict attention to detail will be essential for the success of this experiment. Have ready a small 45°C water bath for prewarming all reagents, as well as a control and an immunized mouse, as assigned.

2. One mouse should be immunized four days ahead of time with 0.2 ml 2% SRBCs injected I.V. (or 0.5 ml injected I.P.). The other mouse will be a nonimmunized control.

3. Prepare two 6-cm Petri dishes by pouring a basal layer of 6 ml 1% Noble agar in balanced salt solution (BSS) and allowing thorough solidification.

4. Prepare 4-ml aliquots of overlayer medium consisting of 0.7% purified agarose in BSS.

5. Kill mice by anesthesia (*not* by cervical separation), and remove spleens. Place each spleen in a 6-cm dish containing 4 ml BSS.

6. With a sharp scalpel, carefully cut through the capsule of each spleen. Gently knead the spleen with a small glass rod (technique will be demonstrated). A milky cell suspension should emanate from the spleen.

7. Place the spleen cell suspension, a tube of 10% SRBC, and a tube containing 4 ml of the overlay medium in the prewarming water bath. Prewarm the basal agar plates to the same temperature.

$$\frac{is}{of} = \frac{x}{100} \qquad \frac{33}{200} = \frac{x}{100}$$

8. Carefully add 0.1 ml 10% SRBCs and 0.2 ml spleen cell suspension to 4 ml overlay. Mix well without introducing air bubbles, and pour onto the previously hardened basal layer of one plate.

9. Allow to harden, and incubate for 1 hr at 37°C.

10. Rinse plate three times with warm (37°C) BSS, 5 min each.

11. Flood plates with 3 ml fresh guinea pig complement diluted 1/7 with BSS.

12. After incubating for 1 hr at 37°C, observe for hemolytic plaques. Confirm microscopically. Plaques should appear as small clear zones encircling single lymphocytes.

Alternative Method

1. Immunize mouse and prepare spleen and SRBC cell suspensions as above.

2. Make Cunningham chambers by placing two strips of double-stick tape 5 cm apart across the short axis of a 1-x-3-in glass slide and placing a second slide on top.

3. Mix 0.5 ml spleen cells with 0.05 ml SRBCs and 0.05 ml fresh, undiluted guinea pig complement. With a capillary pipette, fill the space between the two slides with the suspension without introducing bubbles.

4. Seal the long edges of the slide with molten wax and incubate for 1 hr at 37°C.

5. Score the plaques as above, comparing the results of the immunized and nonimmunized mice.

	Control	*Immune*
Plaque Count		

3. Demonstration of T-Cell Dependent and Macrophage Functions

The T-cell response is characterized by T-cell proliferation and transformation into lymphoblasts. Both antigens and mitogens can induce this response, which also requires the presence of macrophages. Immunologists usually monitor the proliferation by the uptake of a radiolabeled DNA precursor (i.e., ^{3}H-thymidine); however, the response can be followed microscopically by noting the appearance of lymphoblasts in lymphocytes cultured with mitogens. This exercise will demonstrate lymphocyte transformation response to the mitogens, phytohemagglutin (PHA) and concanavalin A (CON-A) in the presence and absence of macrophages.

PROCEDURE

1. Aseptically remove a spleen from a normal mouse, and obtain a spleen cell suspension as described above.

2. Wash three times in 10-ml amounts of BSS by centrifugation at 400 x g for 10 min each.

3. After the last wash, suspend the cells in 10 ml tissue culture fluid (e.g., RPMI-1640).

4. Place 5 ml of this cell suspension in a 6-cm Petri dish, and incubate for 1 hr at 37°C.

5. Place 1 ml of the remaining cell suspension into each of three 12-x-75-mm test tubes. To one tube add 1 ml PHA solution; to another add 1 ml CON-A; and to the third, control tube add 1 ml RPMI-1640.

6. Meanwhile, resuspend and remove the nonadherent cells (i.e., nonmacrophages) from step 4 after the completion of the incubation, and set up three similar tubes as in step 5.

7. Incubate all tubes at 37°C in 5% CO_2 for 3 to 4 days.

8. Remove cells from the incubator, and wash three times in BSS.

9. Resuspend cells from each tube in 0.2- ml aliquots of BSS, and prepare smears on microscope slides.

10. Dry, fix, and stain with Wright's stain.

11. Determine the percentage of lymphoblasts in each slide counting 200 cells in each. Lymphoblasts are recognized as being much larger than lymphocytes, with more abundant cytoplasm and prominent nucleoli. (See FIGURE 5.1.)

FIGURE 5.1. Normal Lymphocyte (A) and Lymphoblast (B)

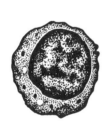
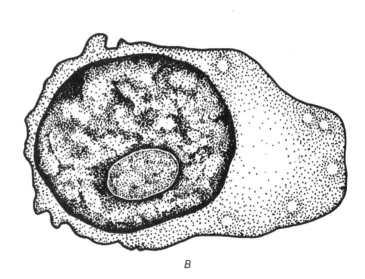

A

B

Mitogen	Total Number of Cells Counted	Number of Immunoblasts	Percent Immunoblasts
PHA			
CON-A			
Control			

Section II

ANTIGEN-ANTIBODY
REACTIONS—SEROLOGY

Exercise 6

AGGLUTINATION

The serological aggregation of particulate antigens by specific antibody is called agglutination. Particulate antigens most commonly employed are erythrocytes, bacteria, or inert particles such as latex or bentonite that have been coated with specific antigen. The aggregation of the particles is due to the formation of a lattice structure between the particles and antibody bridges. Each antibody molecule reacts with two antigenic sites and, if these cites are located on different particles, enough of such reactions will cause a physical aggregation large enough to be visualized. This is the most fundamental serologic reaction, but one which exists in many variations. Red cell and Gram-negative O agglutinins are typically IgM molecules which are probably more efficient due to their size.

This exercise will examine slide and tube methods of agglutination and one of the main features of antigen-antibody reactions, that such reactions are firm and not easily reversible. This property makes it easy to selectively remove antibodies from a mixture by a process of adsorption.

1. Rapid Slide Agglutination

The rapid slide agglutination method is most commonly used for studying the serological aspects of the Gram-negative enteric bacilli and of *Brucella*. For this experiment, any of the commercially available slide agglutination antigens will suffice.

PROCEDURE

1. Using a 0.2-ml pipette graduated in hundredths, pipette the following quantities of antiserum on succeeding rings of an agglutination slide: 0.08, 0.04, 0.02, 0.01, and 0.005 ml.

2. Add to each drop of serum a standardized drop of antigen (0.03 ml). Care must be taken to ensure that the suspension is thoroughly mixed and that the antigen dropper *does not touch* the serum drops.

3. With a clean applicator stick, mix the serum and antigen in the first ring. Break off that portion of the stick moistened by this mixture in order to prevent "carry over" and proceed to the second ring and so on until the contents of all rings have been mixed. The final mixtures of serum and antigen are approximately equal to dilutions of 1/25, 1/50, 1/100, 1/200, 1/500.

4. Immediately after mixing, tilt the agglutination slide back and forth slowly for 2 min.

5. Place the slide in favorable light and observe the results.

6. Record titer: _____ .

2. Tube Agglutination

PROCEDURE

1. Make doubling dilutions of an antiserum to any species of *Salmonella* from 1/20 through 1/10,240 in 0.5-ml quantities. Include a control tube containing 0.5 ml saline.

2. To each tube add 0.5 ml bacterial suspension (1×10^9 organisms/ml) to be tested.

3. Incubation may vary depending on the system under examination but, in general, 3 hr at 45°C followed by overnight in the refrigerator is adequate.

4. If the class is comparing flagellar and somatic agglutinations, place a drop from a tube showing agglutination of each type on a slide and observe microscopically. Are there any differences?

5. If the initial incubation is followed by an overnight storage in the refrigerator, the bacteria will have settled to the bottoms of all tubes. Reading agglutinations is most easily performed with the aid of a magnifying mirror and adequate light. Gently spin the bottom of the tube over the mirror. Agglutination will appear as large clumps or granules in the mirror. Negative tubes will appear as a "wisp of smoke" arising from the bottom of the tube when gently spun.

   Tube agglutination titer of anti- _____ serum: _____ .

3. Agglutination Adsorption

One of the main features of an antigen-antibody reaction is that the combination is a firm and specific one. Therefore, if the antigen is particulate, its corresponding homologous antibodies may easily be removed from a mixture of antibodies. Since the reaction is specific, this facilitates determining the specific antigens or antibodies present in the system, separating the antibodies if two or more kinds are present in the same serum, and concentrating the antibodies in the serum.

PROCEDURE

1. Use an antiserum to *Escherichia coli* for which the titers of the anti-O and anti-B components are known. B antigens are those associated with outer envelope components.

2. To 1 ml of this serum diluted 1/10, add 1 ml of a heavy suspension of a strain of *E. coli* possessing both O and B components.

3. To another 1-ml aliquot of this serum diluted 1/10, add 1 ml of a heavy suspension of *E. coli* in which the B antigen has been removed by heating at 100°C for 1 hr.

4. Incubate both tubes at 40°C to 45°C for 3 hr and then overnight in the refrigerator.

5. Remove the clear supernates with capillary pipettes.

6. Retitrate the adsorbed sera with OB cells, and compare results with the original known values.

   Anti-O titer before adsorption: _____ .
   Anti-B titer before adsorption: _____ .
   Anti-B titer after adsorption with whole cells: _____ .
   Anti-B titer after adsorption with boiled cells: _____ .

4. Bacterial Inagglutinability

Occasionally a known antiserum fails to agglutinate a homologous organism of known antigenic constitution. For instance, certain bacteria containing O antigen may be inagglutinable in a homologous anti-O serum due to the presence of certain other somatic or envelope antigens. Fresh virulent strains of *Salmonella typhosa* often possess a Vi antigen that envelops the cell and thus prevents the O from gaining contact with the corresponding antibody. Likewise, the L, A, and B envelope antigens of *Escherichia coli* may hinder somatic agglutination. The Vi antigen is readily lost on continuous subculture and the envelope antigens of *E. coli* may be removed by various heat treatments.

PROCEDURE

1. Prepare two sets of doubling dilutions in 0.25-ml quantities of an antiserum of *E. coli* containing only the anti-O components.

2. To each tube in the first row add 0.25 ml *E. coli* (1×10^9 organisms/ml) that have previously been heated for 1 hr at 100°C to destroy the B antigen.

3. To each tube in the second row add 0.25 ml of an unheated suspension of *E. coli* OB cells. Mix all tubes thoroughly.

4. Incubate for 3 hr at 45°C, and place in refrigerator overnight.

5. Observe for agglutination. Note titers and explain results.

    Anti-O serum versus O cells: _____ .
    Anti-O serum versus OB cells: _____ .

Exercise 7

ISOIMMUNIZATION

A. HUMAN ISOHEMAGGLUTININS AND ISOHEMAGGLUTINOGENS

Antigens that occur in only certain members of a species and not in others have been demonstrated in the erythrocytes of several species, including man. These isoantigens will stimulate the production of specific isoantibodies when injected into individuals not possessing them. This process of isoimmunization may occur naturally during pregnancy under certain conditions when the fetus possesses isoantigens not present in the maternal circulation or artificially as in the case of blood transfusions. The presence of these antibodies in an individual may result in serious reactions if the corresponding antigens are introduced.

1. Blood Typing

The work of Landsteiner has shown that human blood may be grouped according to what kind of isoantigens they possess. In the most important (ABO) blood grouping system, the type depends on what isoantigen is present on the erythrocytes. Basically, there are two antigens, A and B, which allow four possible blood types—A, B, AB, and O (possessing neither). In this particular blood grouping system, individuals also possess isoantibodies in their sera for the antigen(s) not present in their own circulation (see table below).

A B O Blood Groups

Blood Groups	Isoantigens	Isoantibodies
O	Neither	Anti A and B
A	A	Anti B
B	B	Anti A
AB	A and B	Neither

These antibodies occur naturally in humans shortly after birth, although the antigens have already been determined genetically.

In addition, it has also been shown that there are at least two subgroups of A individuals, designated as A_1 and A_2. This also allows for the individuals with types of A_1B and A_2B.

The ABO antigens are inherited according to Mendelian principles with A and B genes sharing equal dominance over O. As with other inherited traits, different races exhibit different gene frequencies, which results in various distributions of blood types. With this in mind, it can readily be seen how blood group information can be used not only in blood banking and obstetrics, but also in physical anthropology and in certain medico-legal problems, such as cases involving identification of unknown blood stains or disputed parentage.

Determinations of blood groups of the ABO system are rapid and simple. The type is readily ascertained with the aid of known typing sera by the slide agglutination method. Typing sera are prepared in rabbits and are carefully adsorbed so as to be highly specific and not cross-reactive with antigens of other blood grouping systems.

PROCEDURE

1. Using the following typing procedure, type several unknown 5% cell suspensions. After checking your accuracy with the instructor, determine and record your own blood type.

2. Divide a clean microscope slide in two by drawing a line from side to side with a wax pencil.

3. On the right end of the slide, place a drop of known anti-A typing serum; at the opposite end of the slide, place a drop of known anti-B typing serum.

4. At the side of each drop of serum, quickly place drops of the blood to be tested.

5. With one end of an applicatory stick, mix the blood with the anti-A typing sera. Use the other end of the stick to mix the anti-B side of the slide.

6. Continue mixing by tilting the slide back and forth for a few minutes.

7. Reactions are usually strong enough to observe within 5 min. Agglutination or positive reactions will be easily seen by the presence of a granular appearance consisting of large clumps of erythrocytes. Be sure to make observations before drying sets in.

8. Unknown sera may also be typed using known A and B erythrocyte suspensions but the reactions are not as clear-cut. Type several of the unknown sera in this manner.

2. Titration and Adsorption of O Serum

In performing blood transfusions, care must be taken to insure that there is no mixing of incompatible blood. If a recipient's blood contains antibodies for the donor's erythrocytes, a severe reaction may occur to the recipient. Hence, this is the *minimal* criterion of a successful blood transfusion—that the donor's cells must not be agglutinated by the recipient's serum. A table showing compatibilities appears as follows:

Donor's Cells	*Recipient's Serum*			
	A	*B*	*AB*	*O*
A	-	+	-	+
B	+	-	-	+
AB	+	+	-	+
O	-	-	-	-

+ Designates an agglutination reaction

From the above table one can see that considering the ABO system alone, an individual of O type may donate blood to anyone else because the donor's erythrocytes will not be agglutinated by any other serum. Individuals of group O are therefore referred to as "universal donors." However, O serum contains both anti-A and anti-B substances and thus can agglutinate the cells of certain recipients. Ordinarily, for this reason O blood is not used for transfusion to A, B, or AB recipients if compatible blood is on hand. If the anti-A and anti-B titers are not very high, it may be permissible, and indeed even necessary, to use O blood donations since the dilution of these factors upon transfusion will prevent agglutination. It is thus often desirable to know the titer of the anti-A and anti-B substances in O blood for transfusion so that the effect of dilution can be calculated. It is also possible to add specific A and B substances to neutralize these antibodies, resulting in a blood having neither free antigens nor antibody.

PROCEDURE

A. INITIAL ANTI-A AND ANTI-B TITRATIONS

1. Prepare a series of doubling dilutions of O serum from 1/2 through 1/256, using 0.5-ml transfers.

2. Beginning with the highest dilution, transfer 0.2 ml from each dilution to each of two separate tubes. Continue making similar transfers with the next dilution and so on until you have two new rows containing aliquots of each of the original dilutions. In effect you have split the original titration in half.

3. Add 0.2 ml 2% A-cells to each tube in one set and a similar amount of 2% B-cells to each tube in the second set.

4. Include cell-saline controls.

5. Incubate at R°C for 30 min.

6. Centrifuge all tubes at 2000 x g for 2 min.

7. Record titers as the highest dilution that still shows granular clumps of erythrocytes after gentle tapping of the tube.

B. ADSORPTION

1. While the above titrations are being made, each student in a pair should perform an adsorption, one with A, the other with B.

2. To 1 ml of a 1/4 dilution O serum, add 0.5 ml packed, washed erythrocytes.

3. Incubate for 15 min at R°C, and centrifuge at 3000 x g for 3 min.

C. RETITRATION OF ADSORBED SERUM

1. Retitrate the clear supernate as in Part A above from 1/8 through 1/256; divide the titration in two series; add A-cells to one set, B-cells to the other, etc.

2. Record the titers in the table.

Adsorbent	*Titer Versus*	
	A	*B*
None		
A		
B		

3. Compatibility Test—Direct Matching

To insure that there are no antibodies of the saline agglutinating type present in either donor or recipient sera that might result in harmful transfusion reactions, a cross-matching test is necessary. A compatibility or cross-matching test consists of checking donor's serum against recipient's cells and recipient's serum against donor's cells. This is routinely performed before every transfusion. CAUTION: This procedure given below does not rule out all possibilities, such as the Rh "incomplete" antibodies which do not agglutinate in saline. This type of antibody will be discussed in the next experiments.

PROCEDURE

1. Collect the blood from donor and recipient in 5% sodium citrate solution (9 volumes blood to 1 volume 5% sodium citrate). Wash cells three times and make volume of sedimented cells to a concentration of 3% in physiological saline.

2. For serum, collect 20 drops blood from both donor and recipient. After allowing each to clot, centrifuge, and remove the serum.

3. Set up the test as indicated in the table below.

4. Mix all tubes well, and incubate for 30 min at R°C.

5. Centrifuge at 1500 rpm for 3 min.

6. Observe for the presence or absence of agglutination, and record results in the table below.

	Tube Number					
	1	*2*	*3*	*4*	*5*	*6*
Serum of donor	0.25 ml	0.25 ml	—	—	—	—
Serum of recipient	—	—	0.25 ml	0.25 ml	—	—
Cells of donor	—	0.10 ml	0.10 ml	—	0.10 ml	—
Cells of recipient	0.10 ml	—	—	0.10 ml	—	0.10 ml
Saline	0.65 ml	0.65 ml	0.65 ml	0.65 ml	0.90 ml	0.90 ml
Results						

B. THE Rh SYSTEM

The Rh antigen was first described by Landsteiner and Wiener, who showed that rabbits immunized with erythrocytes of *Macacus rhesus* monkeys produced antibodies that agglutinated the erythrocytes of many humans. This discovery probably would not have been important if it had not been recognized that this antigen could give rise to antibodies following transfusions which made subsequent transfusions unsafe. It also has been shown that the hemolytic disease of the newborn (*erythroblastosis fetalis*) is most frequently due to incompatibilities of the Rh system between maternal and fetal blood.

The Rh Antigens

There are two genetic theories proposed for the inheritance of Rh antigens and two corresponding systems of nomenclature. According to Fisher, Rh antigens are inherited by three pairs of genes on adjacent or closely linked loci on the Rh gene-carrying chromosome, each of which determines the production of one of the Rh antigens. The designations of these pairs are C, c; D, d; and E, e. Theoretically, there should be six antisera to react with them. Since each individual chromosome will have three of the possible six Rh genes, the possible chromosome combinations will be eight. The Wiener theory proposes a series of at least eight allelomorphic genes all capable of occupying the *same* locus. They are designated according to the following table:

Fisher	*Wiener*
CDE	R^Z
CDe	R^1
cDE	R^2
cDe	R^O
cdE	r''
Cde	r'
CdE	r^Y
cde	r

This double system of nomenclature has also resulted in two designations of antisera:

Fisher	*Wiener*	*Fisher*	*Wiener*
anti-C	anti-rh'	anti-c	anti-hr'
anti-D	anti-Rh$_O$	anti-d	anti-Hr$_O$
anti-E	anti-rh''	anti-e	anti-hr

Both systems are used in practice, but most students will probably want to stick with the Fisher system.

An antigen for each gene present can be detected in the red cells, if antisera are available. Apparently, the anti-d (anti-Hr$_O$) is unknown and is not available. However, the other five are usually obtainable from most commercial sources.

Since most transfusion isoimmunizations and cases of erythroblastosis fetalis are due to the D(Rh$_O$) antigen (and since this was the one first discovered), individuals bearing this antigen are termed Rh positive. They may be either homozygous or heterozygous. Individuals not possessing the D antigen are obviously homozygous for the d(Hr$_O$) antigen and are termed Rh negative.

In this experiment, the method of determining Rh antigens will be performed. Typing sera are not prepared in rabbits as was the case with the AB antisera, but are obtained from human donors.

4. Rh Tube Test

1. The student should first type for the presence or absence of the D(Rh$_O$) antigen on known positive and negative cells. After verifying the results, the student should type his or her own blood, using as many different antisera as are available.

2. Prepare a 2% suspension of erythrocytes to be studied in physiological saline.

3. Add one drop of commercial antiserum to a small test tube (10-x-75 mm).

4. Add two drops 2% cell suspension.

5. Incubate for 30 min. (Consult manufacturer's directions for correct incubation. Some sera are so strong that an incubation period results in a prozone.)

6. Centrifuge for 1 min at 1000 rpm.

7. Gently agitate the tube, and examine for agglutination.

8. After determining the antigens present, compute your possible genotypes. Knowing the reactions of your parents' erythrocytes will narrow the possibilities down.

The Rh Antibodies

Unlike the ABO system, the corresponding antibodies for the Rh antigens do not occur naturally, but only as the result of isoimmunization. In addition, the antibodies that do occur do not always behave as do the conventional saline agglutinins with which the student is already familiar. The saline agglutinins do occur, but another type of antibody that does not agglutinate in saline is also found very often. If known Rh positive (D+) cells are incubated with these types of antibodies, they are rendered nonagglutinable by positive saline agglutinating serum as the Rh receptor sites have been pre-empted. Such antibodies are termed blocking or incomplete antibodies.

In addition to the blocking demonstration, these antibodies can also be demonstrated if the cells are suspended in their own plasma or some other protein medium such as 22% bovine albumin. Another method consists of pretreating the D erythrocytes with 0.1% trypsin solution. This treatment renders the cells agglutinable, apparently because the Rh antigen resides beneath the stromatal surface of the cell, which is removed by trypsinization.

The most important means of demonstrating "incomplete" antibodies is by the Coombs test. If the erythrocytes are sensitized by incomplete antibodies that are globulins, they can then be agglutinated by antiglobulin serum (Coombs serum). Obviously, antiglobulin serum would have no effect on unsensitized erythrocytes.

The purpose of these experiments is to demonstrate the nature of the Rh antibodies.

5. Rh Antibodies

1. Blocking test

    a. Set up a series of four small (10-x-75-mm) test tubes.

    b. Place 1 drop *slide/tube* anti-D test serum (contains IgG antibodies) into tubes 1 and 2.

    c. Place 2 drops 2% saline suspension of Rh+ cells in tubes 1 and 3, and 2 drops 2% saline suspension of Rh- cells in tubes 2 and 4.

    d. Incubate at 37°C for 15 min, centrifuge at 1000 rpm for 1 min, and observe for agglutination.

    e. Place 1 drop *saline agglutinating* anti-D serum (contains IgM antibodies) into each tube, and repeat step d.

    f. Explain the results.

2. Coombs test

    a. Set up a series of four small (10-x-75-mm) test tubes.

    b. Place 1 drop *slide-tube* anti-D test serum into tubes 1 and 2.

    c. Place 2 drops 2% saline suspension of Rh+ cells in tubes 1 and 3, and 2 drops 2% saline suspension of Rh- cells in tubes 2 and 4.

    d. Incubate 30 min at 37°C, and wash cells three times in 1-ml aliquots of cold saline.

    e. Resuspend sedimented cells after last washing in 1 drop Coombs serum.

    f. Centrifuge at 1000 rpm for 1 min.

    g. Record and explain the results. Re-evaluate the procedure for a compatibility test (p. 44) in light of this knowledge.

3. Protein diluent test

    a. Into each of two tubes, place 2 drops 2% Rh+ cells suspended in 22% bovine albumin.

    b. Place 1 drop *slide/tube* test serum into tube 1.

    c. Incubate at 37°C for 30 min, and centrifuge at 1000 rpm for 3 min.

    d. Carefully observe the difference between the two tubes.

4. Trypsinized cell technique

    a. Washed Rh+ erythrocytes are trypsinized by adding 1.5 ml 0.1% trypsin (Difco 1/250) to each ml of packed red cells. Following a 30-min incubation at 37°C, the cells are again washed three times and resuspended to effect a 2% suspension.

    b. Prepare doubling dilutions of slide test serum from 1/2 to 1/256 inclusive, using 0.1-ml transfers.

    c. Add 0.1 ml 2% trypsinized Rh+ cells to each tube.

    d. Incubate at 37°C for 30 min.

    e. Centrifuge at 1000 rpm for 1 min, and record the titer.

Blocking Test

Reagent	Tube Number			
	1	*2*	*3*	*4*
Slide Test Serum	1 drop	1 drop	—	—
Rh+ RBCs	2 drops	—	2 drops	—
Rh- RBCs	—	2 drops	—	2 drops
RESULTS				
Tube Test Serum	1 drop	1 drop	1 drop	1 drop
RESULTS				

Coombs Test

Reagent	Tube Number			
	1	*2*	*3*	*4*
Slide Test Serum	1 drop	1 drop	—	—
Rh+ RBCs	2 drops	—	2 drops	—
Rh- RBCs	—	2 drops	—	2 drops
INCUBATE AND WASH 3X				
Coombs	1 drop	1 drop	1 drop	1 drop
RESULTS				

Exercise 8

MICROBIAL HEMAGGLUTINATION

Microbial hemagglutination is a phenomenon whereby erythrocytes of a variety of species can be agglutinated through the agency of microorganisms or their products. This agglutination may be effected either directly or indirectly. In direct microbial hemagglutination, the microorganism (bacterial or viral) or soluble by-products thereof, when mixed with the proper erythrocytes, causes them to be agglutinated. The mechanism of this agglutination differs with the organism. The indirect type of hemagglutination involves the "sensitization" of certain animal red cells with soluble antigens and the subsequent agglutination of these sensitized cells by specific antisera. The erythrocyte merely serves as an indicator of an antigen-antibody reaction. In order to be made quite specific, antisera must first be adsorbed with normal unsensitized red cells of the same species as the red cells sensitized. Other particulate substances such as bentonite and latex spheres have been successfully sensitized with antigens and subsequently agglutinated by antisera.

1. Direct—Viral Hemagglutinins and Hemagglutination Inhibition

Certain viruses have the quality of being able to agglutinate the erythrocytes of certain species directly. There are generally two types of viral hemagglutinins, those that are an integral part of the virus particle itself and those that are easily separable from the infective principle by some means such as simple centrifugation. The type that will be carried out in this exercise will be that in which the hemagglutinin is a part of the virus particle.

Virus hemagglutination can be inhibited by specific viral antiserum. It has been shown that viral neutralizing serum also displays hemagglutinin inhibition. Virus, when mixed with specific antibody, results in a noninfectious suspension that will no longer hemagglutinate erythrocytes. The phenomenon is of great practical as well as academic interest since one can diagnose influenza in the absence of virus isolation, by showing a change in hemagglutinin inhibiting antibody in a patient's serum from the acute to the convalescent stage of the disease.

PROCEDURE—Virus Hemagglutination

1. Place 0.5 ml phosphate-buffered saline (pH 7.2 to 7.4) into each of 12 12-x-75-mm serological tubes. (Alternatively, use microtiter method.)

2. Make doubling dilutions of the virus suspension (from EXERCISE 2, 2) using 0.5-ml transfers. The last tube should contain 0.5 ml saline only.

3. Add 0.5 ml 0.25% chicken erythrocyte suspension to each of the tubes. Mix well.

4. Incubate the tubes at room temperature from 30 min to 60 min. Without disturbing the contents of the tubes, carefully observe for evidence of agglutination patterns by holding the rack overhead with the bottoms of the tubes at eye level. Observe the control tube for a negative reaction, which will be a smooth setting of the cells into either a solid round button or ring.

5. Record the highest dilution of virus showing definite agglutination: _____ . This is one unit of virus. In the inhibition test, four units are used. Record the dilution of virus that would contain four units of 0.5 ml _____ ; four units of 0.25 ml _____ .

PROCEDURE—Hemagglutination Inhibition

1. Make doubling dilutions of an anti-influenza serum in 0.25-ml quantities from 1/2 through 1/1024 (ten tubes). Place 0.25 ml saline into each of two more tubes.

2. Add 0.25 ml (diluted to contain four units) virus suspension into each of the serum dilution tubes and into one of the control tubes. Add 0.25 ml saline to the other control tube. Mix well, and incubate at room temperature for 30 min.

3. Add 0.5 ml 0.25% chicken erythrocytes to each tube. Agitate the tubes thoroughly, and incubate at room temperature for 30 to 60 min and observe for hemagglutination. The titer of the antiserum is the highest dilution of serum that completely inhibits hemagglutination by the four units of virus.

   Serum Titer: _____ .

2. Indirect—Passive Hemagglutination

Indirect hemagglutination differs from direct in that the erythrocytes are not agglutinated by the antigen, but are agglutinated by the antibody after the cells have been sensitized with the antigen. The actual mechanism by which antigen becomes nonspecifically adsorbed to the erythrocytes is not well understood. The procedure has many applications and modifications.

PROCEDURE

1. This technique involves treating erythrocytes with $CrCl_3$ in order that protein antigens may sensitize the cells more readily.

2. Have packed sheep or human O+ erythrocytes washed in 0.9% saline (*not* phosphate buffered saline) available.

3. Mix 0.1 ml *freshly* prepared 0.1% $CrCl_3$ and 0.1 ml human globulin at 0.5 mg/ml.

4. *Immediately* add 0.1 ml of the washed, packed erythrocytes.

5. Incubate at room temperature for 4 min.

6. Wash three times in 0.9% saline, and resuspend to a 2% solution.

7. Titrate against an appropriate antiserum beginning at 1/20 dilution by either a microtube method (0.1-ml volumes) or by microtiter equipment.

8. Let cells sediment for 1 hr at room temperature, and read by pattern.

9. Serum Titer: _____ .

Exercise 9

PRECIPITATION

The precipitin reaction occurs when certain soluble antigens are brought in contact with the homologous antibodies. It resembles the agglutination reaction in many ways, differing principally in that precipitin antigens are not particulate, but are proteins or polysaccharides in solution. The precipitin reaction is highly specific and very sensitive, i.e., capable of detecting unknown reagents in dilutions of 1/100,000 to 1/1,000,000 or more.

It is important to bear in mind that antigens used in precipitin reactions are of molecular size and not cellular. For a given mass of antigen, the total surface area varies inversely as the cube of the particle diameter. This means there are comparatively many more receptor sites in soluble antigens. Therefore, it is necessary that a greater concentration of antibody be present for a given amount of such antigens. If the proportion of soluble antigen to antibodies is too great, precipitation will be inhibited, since completion of the lattice formation is hindered by the superfluous antigen molecules in the system. This results in soluble antigen-antibody complexes. For these reasons, the antigen is the reagent that is usually titrated in precipitin tests. The antiserum may be titrated if the antigen is diluted appropriately enough to effect a proper ratio. An alternative procedure is to carefully layer, without mixing, the antigen over the serum so as to form an interface. Diffusion of each reagent will then occur into the other. If the system is appropriate, precipitation will automatically occur at that point in the tube where the proper ratio has been reached.

It is the purpose of these experiments to examine a few of the many facets of precipitation phenomena.

1. Precipitin Analysis

In titrations of precipitating antigen, three general zones of reaction may be observed. The first tubes may show a zone of inhibition due to excess antigen. Next, as the tubes are observed from left to right, it will be noticed that the precipitation increases to a maximum and then begins to decrease. This zone of maximum precipitation is known as the equivalence zone in which the ratio of antigen to antibody is optimal. The zone following this, where the precipitation decreases until no more is discernible, is called the antibody excess zone. If the precipitates are allowed to settle out, the supernates can be tested for excess antigen or antibody by dividing each supernate into two aliquots, adding antigen to one part and antibody to the other, and reincubating the resulting mixtures. It will then be found that excess antigen occurs on the extreme left, as evidenced by precipitation in the tubes to which antibody was added, and excess antibody on the extreme right. The tube or tubes that show the least amount or no excess antigen or antibody in the supernate is the tube or tubes of equivalent proportions.

The procedure is easily adapted to quantitative antibody determinations by simply performing protein analyses on the washed precipitates obtained from the equivalence titration. The completeness of the precipitation of antibody is verified by demonstrating a slight excess of antigen in the supernate. The total protein in the precipitate less the antigen protein at equivalence represents that of the specific antibody. The ratio of antibody to antigen at the equivalence point is then determined and, knowing the molecular weights of the antibody and antigen, the molecular antibody:antigen ratio can be calculated.

PROCEDURE

NOTE: The following technique is quantitative. The student is expected to use the extreme care necessary for any quantitative analysis.

1. Prepare doubling dilutions of antigen in 1-ml quantities through a predetermined equivalence range (a total of five tubes is suggested). The titration should be performed in 10-ml heavy-walled, centrifuge tubes. This step should be performed with extreme care.

2. Add 1 ml saline to a sixth, control tube.

3. Add to each tube, including the control, 1 ml thoroughly clarified, homologous antiserum diluted 1/5.

4. Mix the contents of each tube thoroughly, and incubate at 37°C for 60 min.

5. Note which tube forms a precipitation first. Roughly score the tubes on a 1+ to 4+ basis for amount of precipitation. Note if any tube proceeds beyond a turbid appearance to flocculation.

6. After scoring, incubate in the cold for 48 hr.

7. Centrifuge all tubes in the cold at 3000 x g for 10 min, and carefully decant and *save both* the precipitates and the supernates from the packed precipitate, being careful not to lose any precipitated particles.

Supernate Analysis

8. Quickly carry out precipitin analysis on the supernates for excess antigen or antibody by the following method.

9. Set up two rows of 12-x-75-mm serological tubes with six tubes in each row.

10. Using a calibrated micropipette, carefully remove two 0.25-ml aliquots from the supernate of each tube of the centrifuged precipitates above.

11. Place one aliquot in one tube in each row and proceed similarly through each dilution and the control. When you finish, you should have two identical rows of supernates from the original precipitin titration.

12. To every tube in the first row, add 0.25 ml 1/50 antiserum.

13. To every tube in the second row, add 0.25 ml antigen diluted to equivalence (instructor must predetermine).

14. Incubate for 1 hr at 37°C, then overnight in the cold.

15. Examine the tubes for the presence of precipitate, and look for that dilution not showing any evidence in either tube.

Precipitate Analysis

16. Dissolve the precipitate in each of the centrifuge tubes by adding 10 ml 2% Na_2CO_3 in 0.1 N NaOH. Mix well.

17. Transfer 1-ml samples from each dissolved precipitate to a separate row of the six 10-ml tubes. Place 1 ml of the alkaline solution in a seventh tube for a blank. An eighth tube should contain 1 ml of a standard (e.g., 250 μg/ml rabbit globulin).

18. Add 5 ml alkaline tartrate solution (50 parts 2% Na_2CO_3 in 0.1 N NaOH: 1 part 0.5% $CuSO_4$: 1 part 1% NaK tartrate) to each tube and mix well.

19. Incubate tubes at 37°C for 20 min.

20. Add 0.5 ml phenol reagent diluted 1/2 (Fisher Scientific Co., So-P-24) to each tube, and mix well.

21. After 30 min of color development, read the tubes at 660 μm. Set the spectrophotometer at zero with the blank.

22. Either read the samples on direct concentration mode in reference to the standard, or compare O.D. readings with a standard curve made up from known concentrations of ~~rabbit globulin.~~ bovine serum albumin

23. Multiply all unknown values by 10 (you analyzed only 1 ml of a 10-ml solution) to determine the amount of protein in each precipitate. Subtract any protein found in tube 6 from each value.

24. Record all data in the following table, and perform the indicated calculations.

25. Assuming the molecular weight of the ovalbumin is 42,000 and all of the antibody is 150,000, IgG determine the mole ratios of each reactant by dividing the μg of antigen and antibody completely precipitated at equivalence by the respective molecular weights. Divide the mole ratio of antigen by that of the antibody, and see how close your answer is to 5, the valence of ovalbumin.

Antigen Dilution	Dilution Antigen N	Ppct Total N	Antibody Protein* by Difference	Antibody Protein* Antigen Protein	Tests on Supernate
1/2					
1/4					
1/8					
1/16					
1/32					
1/320					

* Calculations valid only at equivalence.

2. Gel-diffusion Analysis

Since antibodies are not homogeneous and since there may be many antigens present in even the purest preparations, there are several antigen-antibody reactions possible in a single mixture. The gel-diffusion techniques permit the examination of such multiple systems since this technique facilitates the separation of these reactions and since the individual reactants in a system react independently of each other.

In these techniques, gels, usually clarified agar, are used as matrices for combining diffusion with precipitation. The reactants simply diffuse through the gel towards each other and precipitation results when the equivalence points have been reached. A single antigen will give rise to a single line of precipitation in the presence of its homologous antibody. When two antigens are present in a system, each behaves independently of the other. Thus, if several bands of precipitation are evident, there are at least that many antigen-antibody combinations present.

A layer of melted agar is prepared in a Petri dish in the conventional manner. After hardening, holes are cut into the agar so as to form hollow wells. The wells are filled with the appropriate reagents, and the plate is then incubated. The reactions will occur in the agar as bands of precipitation between the antigen and antiserum wells if the dilutions of the reagents have been suitably prepared. An alternative method is to use filter paper discs saturated with the reagents and placed on the surface of the agar in place of the wells. Incubation may be at any temperature, refrigeration being preferred as microbial contamination is inhibited, though this method takes longer.

This technique has infinite applications, but in general they are: (1) to determine the homogeneity of antigen-antibody systems, (2) to enumerate the minimum number of systems present, (3) to follow the purification of an antigenic mixture, and (4) to elucidate the reactions among serologically related antigens. Using the plate method as an example, assume that the center well in FIGURE 9.1 contains the antiserum, and wells 1 and 2 contain samples of the homologous antigen. The resulting precipitation will appear as a continuous line in the form of an angle. There are no spurs at the angle, and this type of reaction is termed a line of identity.

FIGURE 9.1. Reactions of Identity	**FIGURE 9.2. Reaction of Partial Identity**

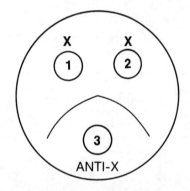 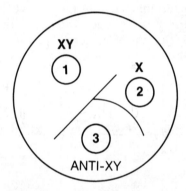

If we place a material in well 1 containing antigenic components X and Y, a material in well 2 containing antigenic component X only, and antiserum in well 3 containing antibodies specific for both X and Y, we will get a reaction similar to that appearing in FIGURE 9.2.

Notice that there is a spur reaction towards the XY well. This indicates that the two antigenic materials are related, but the material in well 1 possesses an antigenic specificity not possessed by the material in well 2. Such a reaction of the formation of a spur indicates partial identity.

If the materials in wells 1 and 2 do not possess common antigens and the antiserum in well 3 possesses specificities for both materials, the reaction will appear as two crossed lines in FIGURE 9.3. If there is no coalescence, the antigens have distinct specificities.

FIGURE 9.3. Reaction of Non-identity

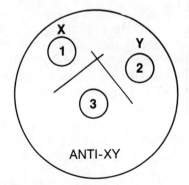

PROCEDURE

1. Pour 6 ml diffusion agar into each of three 60-x-15-mm plastic Petri dishes. The agar may be prepared as follows:

   a. Buffered saline (pH 7.4)   100 ml

   b. Purified agarose   0.8 g

2. Allow the plates to gel thoroughly overnight in the cold before cutting.

3. With an appropriate gel cutter, carefully cut wells into the agar, taking care to cut the gel all the way to the bottom of the dish. If the gel cutter is adjustable, set the wells so that the rims of the outer wells are 7 mm from the rim of the center well.

4. Fill the wells carefully with the designated reagents according to each of the following protocols. Do not overfill.

5. Wait 10 min, and refill wells if necessary.

6. Place plates in a moist chamber, and incubate in the cold for 48 to 72 hr.

7. Record and interpret the reactions by drawing the precipitation lines on the diagrams on the results sheets (FIGURES 9.4, 9.5, and 9.6).

FIGURE 9.4. The Effect of Dilution on Placement of Equivalence Zone

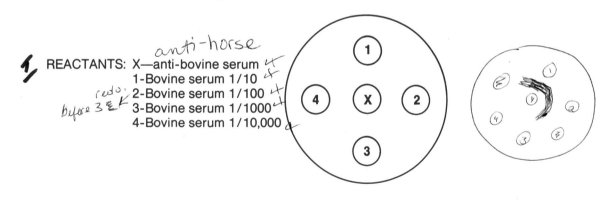

REACTANTS: X—anti-bovine serum
1-Bovine serum 1/10
2-Bovine serum 1/100
3-Bovine serum 1/1000
4-Bovine serum 1/10,000

FIGURE 9.5. Relationship and Composition of Antigens

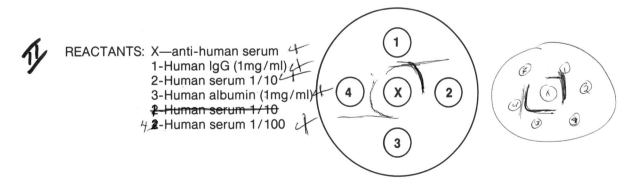

REACTANTS: X—anti-human serum
1-Human IgG (1mg/ml)
2-Human serum 1/10
3-Human albumin (1mg/ml)
2-Human serum 1/10
2-Human serum 1/100

FIGURE 9.6. Relationship of Serologically Related Antigens—Systematic Serology

REACTANTS: X—anti-human serum
1-Human serum 1/10
2-Monkey serum 1/10
3-Human serum 1/100
4-Monkey serum 1/100

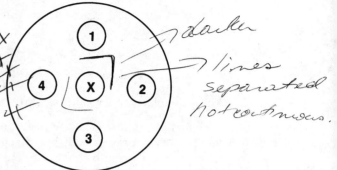

darker
lines
separated
not continuous.

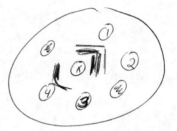

Exercise 10

COMPLEMENT FIXATION

One of the most important nonspecific humoral factors in immunity is a series of substances known as complement. It is present in many species to varying degrees, although in practice, guinea pig serum is usually used as the source since the concentration is more constant and the amount of complement produced is greatest in this species. Complement combines with an antigen *only after the antigen has been sensitized by a specific antibody*. This process is known as complement fixation.

It is important to remember that complement is not a product of an immune reaction but is present in normal sera. Although it is not a single entity and its nature varies among species, some of the following generalizations may be made. Lytic complement is labile to heat, prolonged storage, shaking, and the addition of certain chemicals, such as acids, alkali, ether, bile salts, etc. When it is necessary to destroy the complement activity in a serum, heating at $56°C$ for 20 min is sufficient. This process is termed inactivation and has no effect on most antibodies. At least one IgM or two IgG molecules reacting with an antigen are required to initiate complement activation. IgA does not activate complement by the classical pathway.

The effect of complement activity on the sensitized antigen is usually observed by either lysis or opsonization, depending on the conditions of the system under investigation. If the antigen is cellular, as in the case of erythrocytes, lysis will be the result and is readily observable. If the cellular antigen is bacterial, lysis will occur; however, it is not readily observable except microscopically. If the antigen is soluble or viral in nature, there is no observable result of antigen-antibody union with complement. Nonetheless, complement is fixed in such systems, and the index of this fixation is cleverly demonstrated in the classical complement fixation tests. These procedures employ two antigen-antibody systems: the test system consisting of, first, the specific antigen and antibody in question plus complement, and, second, the indicator system consisting of sheep erythrocytes and rabbit anti-sheep erythrocyte serum (hemolysin). If complement is present at the time of addition of the indicator system, meaning that it was not bound in the original reaction, the erythrocytes will be hemolyzed. If an antigen-antibody reaction had occurred in the initial stage, thus binding the complement, the erythrocytes will not lyse.

In this exercise, we will examine the role of complement in such reactions and become acquainted with the techniques involved in its study.

1. Standardization of Indicator System

To determine the presence of complement-fixing activity of a serum, the serum is incubated with a standardized amount of the homologous antigen in the presence of a standard amount of complement. Following this incubation, it is necessary to determine how much, if any, of the complement was fixed in the initial reaction. This is done by employing the above-mentioned sheep erythrocyte-hemolysin indicator system.

It may readily be seen that such a procedure employing many reagents requires careful controls and standardization. Each reagent must be carefully standardized before the actual complement fixation procedure is carried out. In this experiment, two of the components, complement and the hemolytic sensitizer, will be standardized. One reagent, usually the complement, is held constant while the anti-sheep erythrocyte serum is titrated in its presence. After the standard units of hemolysin are determined, this amount is then held constant while the complement is titrated. This will determine the standard units (usually two) of complement which in the presence of a standard amount (two units) of hemolysin will cause complete lysis of the sheep cells. It will be observed that there is a reciprocal relationship between complement and hemolysin. As the quantity of complement is increased, there is a corresponding decrease in the amount of hemolysin necessary, and vice versa. The important thing is that these two reagents be in balance for use in complement fixation procedures.

A. TITRATION OF HEMOLYSIN

PROCEDURE

> NOTE: It is important that all saline used in the study of complement be supplied with magnesium ions. Dissolve 0.1 g $MgSO_4$ per liter of fresh physiological saline. This will be used in some of the following experiments in this exercise and will hereafter be referred to as Mag saline.

1. Arrange twelve 13-x-100-mm serological tubes in a rack. *2 gtps ① 1/1000 ② 1/100*

2. Prepare a 1/1000* dilution of hemolysin by placing 4.5 ml Mag saline in a test tube and adding 0.5 ml stock 1/100 dilution of hemolysin. Stopper and mix thoroughly.

3. Pipette 0.5 ml 1/1000 hemolysin into each of the first five tubes and into tube 11.

4. Proceed as follows, adding the prescribed amount of saline *buffer* (see column 2) to each tube first:

Tube Number	Mag Saline ml	Process	Final Dilution
1 *hemolysis*	None	None	1/1000
2 *hemolys*	0.5	Mix; discard 0.5 ml	1/2000
3	1.0	Mix; transfer 0.5 ml to tube 6; discard 0.5 ml	1/3000
4	1.5	Mix; transfer 0.5 ml to tube 7; discard 1.0 ml	1/4000
5	2.0	Mix; transfer 0.5 ml to tube 8; discard 1.5 ml	1/5000
6	0.5	Mix; transfer 0.5 ml to tube 9	1/6000
7	0.5	Mix; transfer 0.5 ml to tube 10	1/8000
8	0.5	Mix; discard 0.5 ml	1/10,000
9	0.5	Mix; discard 0.5 ml	1/12,000
10	0.5	Mix; discard 0.5 ml	1/16,000

no hemolysis

11 *no hemolysis*   12 *no hemolysis.*

5. Add 0.3 ml 1/30* fresh guinea pig complement into each of the first ten tubes and into tube 12.

6. Add 1.7 ml Mag saline to the first ten tubes, 2 ml to tube 11, and 2.2 ml to tube 12.

7. Add 0.5 ml 2% suspension of sheep erythrocytes to each tube. Mix the contents of all tubes thoroughly.

8. Incubate in a 37°C water bath for 30 min.

* The initial dilutions of hemolysin and complement may have to be determined by a preliminary rough titration.

9. The unit of hemolysin is the highest dilution that gives complete hemolysis. The complement fixation test employs two units of hemolysin to ensure an adequate excess. Be sure to inspect the controls to ensure reliability of the reagents.

ex· 1/800

One unit of hemolysin: ___1/2000___ dilution in 0.5 ml

Two units of hemolysin: ___1/1000___ dilution in 0.5 ml

1/400

B. TITRATION OF COMPLEMENT

PROCEDURE

1. While the above titration is being carried out, the complement titration may be prepared.

2. Place eleven 13-x-100-mm tubes in a rack.

3. Beginning with tube 1, add 0.1 ml 1/30 complement, 0.15 ml to tube 2, 0.2 ml to tube 3, and so on through tube 9, increasing the amount by 0.05 ml with each succeeding tube. Add 0.5 ml 1/30 complement to tube 10.

4. At this point, certain procedures, e.g., Kolmer, require the addition of antigen in 0.5-ml quantities followed by enough Mag saline to effect final volume of 2 ml. This is then incubated from 30 to 60 min to take into consideration any nonspecific binding of complement. The hemolysin and sheep cells are added next and the tubes reincubated in a 37°C water bath for 30 min. An alternate procedure (which does not take into consideration nonspecific binding) omits the addition of antigen and proceeds directly to the hemolysin as in the next step.

5. Add two units of hemolysin contained in 0.5 ml (dilution as determined in the preceding titration) to each of the first nine tubes and 0.5 ml to tube 11.

6. Add enough Mag buffer saline (see chart below) to effect a final volume of 2 ml in each tube.

7. Add 0.5 ml 2% suspension of sheep erythrocytes to each tube. Mix the contents of each tube thoroughly.

Tube Number	Complement 1/30	Hemolysin 2 units	Mag Saline	2% SRBC
1 no hemolysis	0.1 ml	0.5 ml	1.4 ml	0.5 ml
2 not complete	0.15 ml	0.5 ml	1.35 ml	0.5 ml
3 complete	0.2 ml	0.5 ml	1.3 ml	0.5 ml
4 complete	0.25 ml	0.5 ml	1.25 ml	0.5 ml
5 complete	0.3 ml	0.5 ml	1.2 ml	0.5 ml
6 no hemolysis	0.35 ml	0.5 ml	1.15 ml	0.5 ml
7	0.4 ml	0.5 ml	1.1 ml	0.5 ml
8	0.45 ml	0.5 ml	1.05 ml	0.5 ml
9	0.5 ml	0.5 ml	1.0 ml	0.5 ml
10 no hemolysis	0.5 ml	—	1.5 ml	0.5 ml
11 no hemolysis	—	0.5 ml	1.5 ml	0.5 ml

8. Incubate in a 37°C water bath for 30 min.

9. Determine the smallest amount of complement giving *complete* lysis. This is the *exact* unit. The *full* unit is 0.05 ml more than the *exact* unit. For use in the complement fixation tests,

complement is diluted so that *two full* units are contained in 1 ml. Compute the dilution necessary so that the complement you have standardized will contain two full units per milliliter as balanced against two units of hemolysin.

ex

Exact unit: _____ 2 _____ ml of 1/30 complement · 3 ml

Full unit: _____ .25 _____ ml of 1/30 complement · 35 ml.

Two full units: _____ .50 _____ ml of 1/30 complement .35^2 = .7

Dilution necessary to contain two full units/ml: _____ 1/60 _____

30 → dilution

$\frac{30}{.7}$ $\frac{30}{.5}$ $\frac{1}{60}$ $\frac{60}{.5\overline{)30.0}}$ $\frac{30}{.7} = \frac{1}{43}$

2. Anticomplementary Effects

Many sera and antigens have the ability of nonspecifically removing or inactivating complement by themselves. This anticomplementary effect must be eliminated or, if it cannot be eliminated, must be determined. Reagents that have particulate matter in them, are microbially contaminated, or contain certain agents such as soap tend to be anticomplementary. In the case of sera, this effect is usually removed by heating at 56°C for 30 min immediately before testing. This procedure is necessary anyway to inactivate the complement present in any fresh serum. Antigens must be titrated in the presence of complement to determine what value is safe to use in the test.

PROCEDURE

The procedure for determining the anticomplementary effect of the serum (providing it cannot be removed by heating) is easily accomplished by making doubling dilutions of the serum in 0.2-ml quantities, adding two full units (1 ml) of complement and 0.5 ml Mag saline to each dilution, and incubating for 30 min at 37°C. Following the incubation, hemolysin and sheep cells are added to every tube and reincubated. The anticomplementary value is the largest quantity of serum that, in the absence of antigen, does not interfere with the activity of complement.

The procedure for determining the anticomplementary action of an antigen is carried out in the same manner, except that antigen dilutions are made in 0.5-ml quantities. The anticomplementary value of the antigen is the largest amount that, in the absence of specific antibodies, does not interfere with the action of complement.

3. Determination of Antigenic Dose

It is very important that a standard reactive dose of antigen be employed in complement fixation tests. The dose should not be hemolytic or anticomplementary. It should be specific, resulting in complete binding of complement in the presence of a known positive serum, and it should be sensitive enough to detect minute quantities of antibodies. The dose is most easily determined by performing a "checkerboard" titration in which several dilutions of antigen are concurrently titrated against successive dilutions of a known strongly positive serum.

PROCEDURE

1. Prepare a master titration of antigen through six doubling dilutions (1/40 through 1/1280 for Kolmer antigens) in 3-ml quantities.

2. Prepare a master titration of a strongly positive antiserum through five doubling dilutions (1/5 through 1/80 for sera used in Kolmer tests) in 2-ml quantities.

3. Arrange five rows of 13-x-100-mm test tubes with six tubes in each row.

4. Pipette antigen as follows:

> Tube 1 of each row—0.5 ml 1/40 antigen
> Tube 2 of each row—0.5 ml 1/80 antigen
> Tube 3 of each row—0.5 ml 1/160 antigen
> Tube 4 of each row—0.5 ml 1/320 antigen
> Tube 5 of each row—0.5 ml 1/640 antigen
> Tube 6 of each row—0.5 ml 1/1280 antigen

5. Pipette serum dilutions as follows:

> Add 0.2 ml 1/5 serum to each tube in the first row
> Add 0.2 ml 1/10 serum to each tube in the second row
> Add 0.2 ml 1/20 serum to each tube in the third row
> Add 0.2 ml 1/40 serum to each tube in the fourth row
> Add 0.2 ml 1/80 serum to each tube in the fifth row

6. Add 1 ml complement (two units) to each tube. Some procedures such as the Kolmer require a 15-min incubation before the addition of complement.

7. Prepare the following controls:

   a.   Serum control—0.2 ml 1/5 serum
   > 1.0 ml complement (two units)
   > 0.5 ml Mag saline

   b.   Antigen control—0.5 ml antigen 1/40
   > 1.0 ml complement (two units)
   > 0.2 ml Mag saline

   c.   Hemolytic system control—1.0 ml complement (two units)
   > 0.7 ml Mag saline

8. The incubation period varies depending on the nature of the system under examination. The Kolmer test requires 15 to 18 hr in the refrigerator, but incubation in a 37°C water bath for 30 to 60 min is adequate for most purposes. If refrigerator incubation is used, place tubes in a 37°C water bath for 10 min before proceeding to the next step.

9. After incubation, add 0.5 ml hemolysin (two units) and 0.5 ml 2% suspension of sheep erythrocytes to each tube.

10. Mix the contents of each tube well, and incubate at 37°C for 30 min.

11. Record results in the table provided. Be sure to inspect the controls first. The dose of antigen to be employed in the test is the largest amount giving 4+ fixation with the smallest amount of serum.

	Antigen Dilutions					
Serum Dilutions	*1/40*	*1/80*	*1/160*	*1/320*	*1/640*	*1/1280*
1/80						
1/40						
1/20						
1/10						
1/5						

Antigenic dose: _____ .

4. Wassermann-Kolmer Test

The Wassermann-Kolmer test is used as a supplement in the diagnosis of syphilis. Much that is known about complement fixation has come about through the study of this test. The antigen used in this test is an alcoholic extract of cardiolipin from beef heart. Although this is a heterogenetic antigen, it demonstrates a very high degree of specificity for antibodies produced in syphilitics. The Wassermann antigen is a hapten i.e., it is capable of reacting with antibody, but it is not capable of stimulating their production.

It has already been observed that rigid standardization is necessary before performing the complement fixation test proper. Rigid controls are also important to ensure that the many variables are behaving properly. Conventionally, the Wassermann-Kolmer test consists of 11 tubes; the first of these represents the test proper and the rest represent the controls. If many sera are being tested at once, only one set of controls (except for the unknown serum control) is necessary. The student should be familiar with the purpose of each control before beginning this experiment.

In recent years, the use of the Reiter strain of *Treponema pallidum* as the antigen has been instituted for the complement fixation diagnosis of syphilis. Although the actual pathogen of syphilis appears to be an obligate parasite, the Reiter strain is easily cultivated on thioglycollate broth containing 10% bovine or swine serum. The complement fixation procedure using the Reiter antigen is much the same as that of the Wassermann-Kolmer technique and is much more specific.

PROCEDURE

1. Set up eleven 13-x-100-mm test tubes according to the following table.

2. Incubate the fixation stage in the refrigerator for 15 to 18 hr.

3. After incubation, warm the tubes in a 37°C water bath for 10 min, add the prescribed amount of hemolysin and 2% sheep erythrocytes, and reincubate for 30 min at 37°C. Record results immediately after the last incubation period.

4. Each student will be given several samples of unknown sera, one sample of known positive serum, and one sample of known negative serum for examination.

The Wassermann-Kolmer Test

Tube No.	Name	Serum	Antigen	Complement 2 Units	Mag Saline	Hemolysin 2 Units	2% SRBC	Results
1	Unknown Serum	0.2 ml	0.5 ml	1 ml	—	0.5 ml	0.5 ml	
2	Positive Serum	0.2	0.5	1	—	0.5	0.5	
3	Negative Serum	0.2	0.5	1	—	0.5	0.5	
4	Unknown Serum Control	0.2	—	1	0.5	0.5	0.5	
5	Positive Serum Control	0.2	—	1	0.5	0.5	0.5	
6	Negative Serum Control	0.2	—	1	0.5	0.5	0.5	
7	Antigen Control	—	0.5	1	0.2	0.5	0.5	
8	Hemolytic System Control	—	—	1	0.7	0.5	0.5	
9	Complement Control	—	—	1	1.2	—	0.5	
10	Hemolysin Control	—	—	—	1.7	0.5	0.5	
11	Cell Saline	—	—	—	2.2	—	0.5	

5. CH$_{50}$ Determination

Often is it necessary to measure the amount of hemolytic complement in a serum. In certain chronic inflammatory diseases and complement deficiency syndromes, the value may be abnormally low. Experimentally, it is occasionally informative to measure the total hemolytic complement activity in a serum before and after incubating a serum in the presence of an activator to see how much complement is consumed by the activation.

Measurement of complement is expressed in CH$_{50}$ units (i.e., that amount of complement in a given volume of serum capable of lysing 50% of the sensitized sheep erythrocytes in a test system). Sheep erythrocytes (E) are first incubated with antibody (A) to prepare sensitized erythrocytes (EA) and these are simply mixed with a *fresh* sample of the test serum. Results are plotted on probit paper and the CH$_{50}$ value determined.

If time is limited and only one complement experiment can be performed, it is suggested that this one be used. If the EA are prepared ahead of time, the test can be completed well within a 2-hr laboratory period.

PROCEDURE

1. The following reagents should be prepared first:

    a. Veronal* buffered saline (VBS) 5X with metals (Me^{++})

NaCl	83.0 g
Sodium diethyl barbiturate*	10.19 g
1 N HCl	34.6 ml
Stock Mg^{++} and CA^{++} solution	5 ml
(MgCl$_2$ · 6H$_2$O - 20.33 g and CaCl$_2$ · 2H$_2$O 4.4 g in 100 ml distilled water)	
Distilled water	q.s. ad 2000 ml

    Dilute 1/5 before use; adjust pH to 7.2.

    b. 5X VBS without Me^{++}

    Same as above, but Minus Ca^{++} and Mg^{++}.

    c. 0.15 M Na$_2$EDTA

    5.58 g/100 ml H$_2$O, adjust pH to 7.4.

    d. 0.01 M EDTA-VBS buffer

    40 ml 5X VBS without Me^{++}
    13.3 ml 0.15 M Na$_2$EDTA   MAKE FRESH EACH DAY!
    q.s. ad to 200 ml   DO NOT KEEP!

2. Preparation of E:

    a. Wash 5 ml SRBC once with 1X VBS with Me^{++}.

    b. Wash 2X with EDTA-VBS buffer.

    c. Resuspend to 8 ml EDTA-VBS buffer if you know hemolysin titer; VBS with Me^{++} if not.

    d. Place 0.2 ml in 4.8 ml *water* and read at 541 mμ. Blank with plain water.

---

* See Appendix for substitute for barbiturates.

e. $\dfrac{\text{O.D. at 541}}{0.420}$ X Volume to be adjusted = Corrected volume

f. Adjust SRBCs or E to corrected volume.

3. Determination of A or hemolysin titer (use VBS with Me^{++} throughout):

a. Titer hemolysin in 0.5-ml quantities from 1/50 to 1/6400.

b. Add 0.5 ml adjusted E to each tube. Mix well.

c. Incubate at 37°C for 20 min.

d. Spin and wash 1X in VBS.

e. Add 1 ml 1/100 commercial guinea pig complement to each tube.

f. Add 6.5 ml VBS to each tube. Mix well.

g. Incubate 90 min at 37°C.

h. Centrifuge, read at 541 mμ, and plot O.D. versus dilution of hemolysin. It is desirable to select a dilution of hemolysin for use in the determination so that extra hemolysin will not appreciably alter the amount of lysis, yet will still be in slight excess. Select a dilution on that part of the curve that plateaus. An ideal situation is depicted in the graph in FIGURE 10.1.

FIGURE 10.1 Ideal Hemolysin Dilution Graph

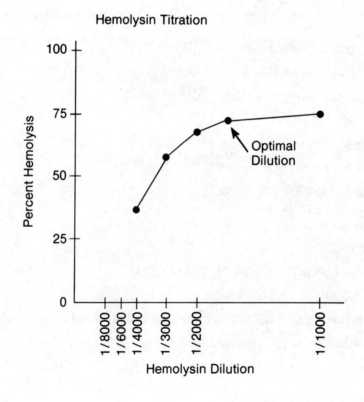

4. Preparation of EA:

    a. Mix equal volumes of E in EDTA-VBS buffer and hemolysin, diluted in EDTA-VBS.

    b. Incubate at 37°C for 20 min; centrifuge.

    c. Wash 1X in EDTA buffer and 2X in VBS with Me^{++}.

    d. Resuspend final cell pellet in a volume $\cong$ 3X or 4X original cell volume of EA (as in 4a) in VBS with Me^{++}.

    e. To 0.2 ml of this, add 4.8 ml *water*, read at 412 mμ. Optimum O.D. = *0.60*. Adjust if necessary.

5. Test Proper:

    a. Add 0.6 ml EA to each of five tubes/determination.

    b. Dilute 0.1 ml human sample + 2.4 ml VBS. (This dilution varies with the operator. It will be necessary to have three points that are plottable below. One may have to alter this dilution in order to achieve the three points. If rabbit serum is used, dilute 0.2 ml of serum with 2.8 ml of VBS.)

    c. To the EA tubes, add increasing amounts of diluted sample (i.e., 0.6, 0.4, 0.3, 0.2, and 0.1).

    d. Now add 2.8, 3.0, 3.1, 3.2, and 3.3 ml VBS, respectively.

    e. Mix well and incubate 60 min at 37°C; mix at 20 min and 40 min.

    f. Centrifuge 3 min, full speed.

    g. Read supernate at 550 mμ "zeroed in" against a VBS blank.

    h. Control is used to set at 100% and consists of 0.6 ml EA + 3.4 ml *water*.

    i. Calculate percent lysis = O.D. of unknown/O.D. 100% water control.

    j. Plot percent lysis versus volume on probit paper provided (FIGURE 10.2).

    k. Calculate CH$_{50}$ according to:

$$\frac{\text{Dilution used (25 for human; 15 for rabbit)}}{50\% \text{ value obtained from plot on probit paper}} = CH_{50}$$

6. The Alternative Pathway

The preceding experiments have all been done by activating the classical complement pathway by immune complexes. In addition to this pathway, several mechanisms of activating the alternative pathways have become well recognized. Although immune complexes can also activate the alternative pathway, many substances are known that activate this pathway nonspecifically (i.e., in the absence of antibody). Materials such as inulin, zymosan, and bacterial lipopolysaccharide are well-known, nonspecific alternative pathway activators. In the alternative pathway, the early cascade components (C1, C2, and C4) are bypassed and C3 is activated by a variety of means.

Two well-known means of detecting alternative pathway activation are by differential chelation and immunoelectrophoresis. In the former, two chelating agents, ethylene diamine tetraacetate (EDTA) and ethylene glycol tetraacetate (EGTA), are added to separate tubes containing the activator and a known amount of complement. EDTA will inhibit both the classical and alternative pathways since it ties up magnesium and calcium ions, both essential cations for complete activation. On the other hand, EGTA in the presence of supplementary magnesium inhibits only the classical pathway and not the alternative, owing to its selective chelation of calcium. The other common way in which the alternative pathway is detected is by the immunoelectrophoretic demonstration (see EXERCISE 14, 2) of conversion of a C3 proactivator (factor B) to its active form (Bb). The purpose of this experiment is to demonstrate nonspecific complement activation by the alternative pathway.

PROCEDURE

1. To three 0.5-ml amounts of fresh human, guinea pig, or rabbit serum, add 0.1 ml saline containing 1 mg inulin.

2. Set up a fourth control tube containing 0.5 ml serum and 0.1 ml saline.

3. To one of the inulin-serum tubes, add 25 μl 0.1 M disodium EDTA.

4. To the additional inulin-serum tube, add 25 μl MgEGTA (see Appendix for formulation).

5. To the third inulin-serum tube and the saline control, add 25 μl saline.

6. Incubate at 37°C for 30 min.

7. Centrifuge at 2500 rpm for 5 min. Remove and save supernates.*

8. Add 40 μl 0.1 M $CaCl_2$ to each tube containing EDTA or MgEGTA (to reverse chelation) and 40 μl saline to the others.

9. Assay all four fractions for CH_{50} as in previous experiment. (Lower dilutions than recommended may be necessary in those tubes where complement activation is expected.)

10. Explain the observed results.

---

* It is suggested that this experiment be run with human serum in conjunction with Immunoelectrophoresis (EXERCISE 14, 2). Electrophorese samples and develop with anti-human factor B. Examine the slides for the appearance of one (unactivated) or two (activated) precipitin arcs.

FIGURE 10.2. Lysis Probit Graph Paper

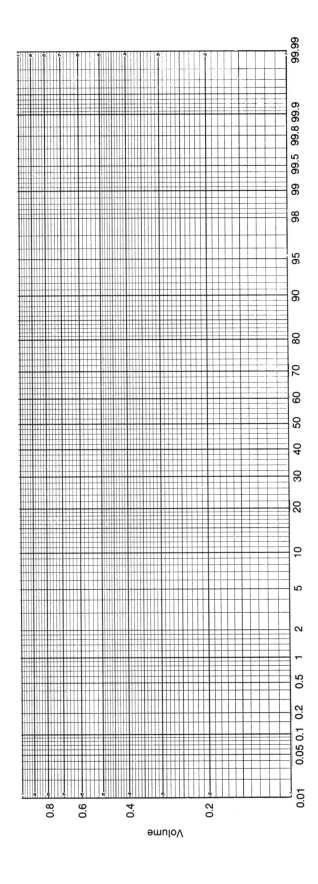

Exercise 11
ELISA

Primary antigen-antibody reactions such as agglutination and precipitation are excellent tools for rapid serologic determinations, but are limited in the sensitivity that can be achieved by them. Under the best of circumstances, such primary methods can detect as little as 1 to 100 ng of antibody N. When one labels the antibody, or in some cases the antigen, with radioisotopes, fluorescent dyes, or enzymes, using the correct technology one can extend the sensitivity of serological reactions to the picogram level and beyond.

These secondary types of serological reactions are exemplified in this experiment by the enzyme-linked immunoadsorbent assay or ELISA. In this instance, a protein antigen is physically adsorbed to plastic microtiter wells before reacting with antiserum dilutions.

After reacting with antiserum, the wells are washed, and the reactions developed by adding an antiglobulin to which a given enzyme has been conjugated. Following addition of an appropriate substrate for this enzyme, a visible color reaction in the enzyme modified substrate is recorded optically. Such a reaction will only occur in those wells that have bound the enzyme-linked antiglobulin, which in turn has bonded with the primary antigen-antibody complex.

PROCEDURE

1. It will be important to use the correct buffer as several different ones will be used in this experiment.

2. Coat ten wells in a row of a plastic microtiter plate with ovalbumin diluted to a concentration of 10 μg/ml dissolved in *Coating* buffer. Each well should receive 100 μl. Skip well 11 and add 100 μl of the antigen to well 12.

3. In a second row, fill similar wells with 100-μl quantities of *Coating* buffer to serve as blanks.

4. Incubate for 30 min at 37°C.

5. While the plates are incubating, titrate an anti-ovalbumin serum beginning at 1/50 through ten dilutions in 0.25-ml quantities. Titrate the serum in *Diluting* buffer with a micropipette.

6. Wash the plates carefully using a well washing device (e.g., Nunc Immunowash) designed to wash all wells in a row at a time. This must be done at least eight times using *Wash* buffer. Remove all buffer after the last wash.

7. Beginning with the last serum dilution, transfer 100 μl to well 10 of each row; then move to the next serum dilution and similarly transfer 100 μl to well 9 of each row and so on until you have reached the starting dilution, 100 μl of which should be transferred to each well 1.

8. Incubate for 30 min at 37°C.

9. Wash all wells as in step 6 with *Wash* buffer.

10. Add 100 μl of commercial goat anti-rabbit globulin conjugated to horseradish peroxidase (diluted 1/500 in *Diluting* buffer) to every well.

11. Incubate for 30 min at 37°C and then wash.

12. Add 100 μl of peroxidase substrate in freshly prepared *Substrate* buffer to each well.

13. Incubate at room temperature for 30 min and read the plates visually on a 1+ to 4+ basis or at 540 μm if a microtiter plate reader is available. Set the optical density of the instrument to zero with the antigen control (well 12 in the first row). Subtract any O.D. in the antibody controls (bottom row) from the corresponding test well above. Record the results in the table below.

	1	2	3	4	5	6	7	8	9	10	12
Ab											
Ctrl											

Section III

IMMUNOCHEMISTRY

Immunochemistry, as the name indicates, is the study of the chemistry of immune reactions, antigens, and antibodies employing the precise analytical methods of chemisty and the highly specific reactions of immunology. Although this subject is not new, there have been many recent advances that have made great contributions not only to immunology, but also to the study of proteins, enzymes, polysaccharides, embryology, and systematics.

Many of the tools and techniques of the immunochemist are very specialized, requiring highly trained individuals to use them adequately. Nevertheless, some of the more basic and important concepts and techniques are included in this section to acquaint the beginning student with this fascinating field.

Exercise 12

GEL FILTRATION

One of the most powerful tools in biochemical and immunochemical technology is the technique of molecular sieving or gel filtration. In this process, a bed of particles of highly cross-linked polysaccharide polymers of neutral charge serves as a molecular sieve. The pore size of this material is carefully regulated so that only molecules of a certain molecular weight range can enter the gel particles while heavier weight molecules are excluded from the pores of the particles and wash on through the column. If beads of polymers with a pore size admitting molecules with a molecular weight of 200,000 or less are used to separate serum proteins, IgM molecules are excluded and pass immediately through the column in a volume of eluting fluid (e.g., saline), equal to the volume of the bed of the gel. IgG molecules, being less than 200,000 molecular weight, enter the pores and remain there until this volume of eluting fluid has passed through the column, after which time they begin to elute.

In addition to its use in separating immunoglobulins, gel filtration is also most useful in desalting fractionated protein solutions (use of a gel with a small pore size) and in separating various antigens from mixtures on the basis of size. It is the method of choice of separating polysaccharide macromolecules, which often are of neutral charge and thus cannot be attracted to ion exchange resins. The useful thing about a properly prepared gel filtration column is that it can be used over and over as almost all materials can be easily washed from the column. An unfortunate exception is fluorescein isothiocyanate, a dye commonly used in immunohistochemistry. If certain gels are used to separate bound from unbound dye, the gel will have to be discarded as the unbound dye irreversibly binds to the gel.

1. Desalting Precipitated Globulins

PROCEDURE

1. Prepare 1 liter of physiological saline from freshly boiled distilled water. Allow to cool to R°C.

2. It will first be necessary to prepare the gel for packing the columns by allowing the beads to swell sufficiently. The table below lists a few of the gels available under the trade name Sephadex, their approximate exclusion limits, the amount of water necessary to add to each gram of dry gel, and the length of time required to allow the gel to swell at room temperature.

Gel	Exclusion Limit	Water Regain/g	Minimum Swelling Time
G-25	5000	4-6	3 hr
G-50	10,000-30,000	9-11	3 hr
G-100	100,000-150,000	15-20	72 hr
G-200	200,000-800,000	30-40	72 hr

3. For this experiment, allow 20 g G-25 Sephadex to swell for at least 3 hr in 300 ml saline.

4. Remove dissolved air from the suspension by degassing under gentle vacuum (water aspirator) for 15 min.

5. Mount a column approximately 2.5 cm wide and high enough to contain a bed 30 to 50 cm in length. The dead space at the bottom of the column should be as small as possible (e.g., not more than 0.1% of bed volume). It is important to mount the column exactly vertical.

6. Equip the column outflow with a small piece of tubing that can be regulated with a screw clamp.

7. Pour a small amount of degassed saline into the column, and allow some to run out of the tubing to displace the air.

8. Pour the degassed slurry into the column by means of a glass rod, and allow to settle. If air channels form, it will be necessary to repack the column.

9. Check to make sure the top of the bed is even and level. The height of the bed volume should be at least ten times its width.

10. Set up a reservoir of eluting fluid (saline) connected to the column by means of small-bore tubing. The height differential between the reservoir fluid height and the end of the column outlet tubing should not be more than 15 cm.

11. Allow two to three bed volumes of saline to pass through the column.

12. Place 5 ml serum in a heavy-walled centrifuge tube immersed in an ice bath.

13. After the serum has chilled, add slowly with constant stirring an equal volume of saturated $(NH_4)_2SO_4$. Stopper the tube, and place in an ice bath overnight.

14. Centrifuge at 3000 g for 5 to 10 min and discard supernate. Wash the precipitated globulin three times in cold half-saturated $(NH_4)_2SO_4$ in the same manner.

15. Dissolve percipitate in as little distilled water as possible. A clear but opalescent solution will result.

16. Carefully remove eluant above bed volume by suction or by draining. Care should be taken to never allow bed to go dry.

17. Gently layer sample onto bed by means of a capillary pipette. Open the column outlet and allow the sample to completely enter the bed, but not to drain below bed surface. Close column outlet.

18. Gently wash sides of column with 2 to 3 ml saline, and allow this to enter column.

19. Without mixing the resin, carefully fill column with saline, and connect to reservoir. Open column outlet, and commence the run.

20. The progress of the protein through the column can be visually followed by means of ultraviolet light. As the protein nears the column outlet or after a volume of eluant has passed through the column equal to the bed volume, begin checking elution drops with drops of saturated $(NH_4)_2SO_4$.

21. Begin collecting eluant immediately after the first precipitation forms. The sample will become diluted approximately twofold as it passes through the column. When this volume is reached or when elution drops contain no more protein as determined by the $(NH_4)_2SO_4$ test, cease collection, but continue to pass eluant through column.

22. After a brief interval, the $(NH_4)_2SO_4$ will be eluted. Continue passing another bed volume of saline through the column or enough saline that the eluant no longer precipitates with a 10% $BaCl_2$ solution.

23. The protein solution may then be used for further experiments free of excessive salt concentration.

2. Immunoglobulin Separation

PROCEDURE

1. Using the principles above, prepare a 1.5-cm column with Sephadex G-200 (allow 1 g of resin to swell for three days in 200 ml saline to which sodium azide has been added to effect a 0.02% concentration). Degas and pack column.

2. The operating pressure on this resin is more critical and should be carefully observed. Apply a 0.5-ml sample of a serum containing known IgM red cell agglutinins.

3. Adjust flow rate of column to equal about 7 ml/hr. The collection of samples from such a flow rate will require the use of an automatic fraction collector set to collect 0.5 ml or 10-drop aliquots.

4. If the fraction collector is equipped with an ultraviolet absorption monitor, an elution curve can be constructed from the readout. Otherwise read each aliquot at 280 mμ and plot absorbance versus fraction number or elution volume.

5. Pool those tubes occurring under each peak and either titrate against specific red cells or assay by means of immunoelectrophoresis (*vide infra*).

Exercise 13

CHROMATOGRAPHY

The resins used in ion exchange chromatography differ in that the polymers are highly charged and do not consist of pores. Materials passing through a column made up of such materials are selectively adsorbed according to the relative charge density of each constituent. Columns prepared from charged cellulose resins may be cation exchangers (carboxymethyl or CM-cellulose) or anion exchangers (DEAE-cellulose). When serum is added to a DEAE column, acidic proteins such as those found in serum are adsorbed immediately. Next a stepwise or gradient elution of the proteins is carried out by modifying the solute concentration or the pH of the eluting buffer sequentially. As the molarity of the buffer increases, there will be an increasing affinity of and competition by the buffer salts for the adsorbent. The IgG molecules and others with low net charge are thus eluted first as the buffer concentration increases. These will be followed in order by molecules of increasing net charge. Size may also play a role in that molecules of larger size, but with the same net charge density per unit surface area, may be eluted later than smaller molecules. This explains why IgM molecules come off the column later than IgA.

1. DEAE Ion Exchange Chromatography

PROCEDURE

1. Solutions

    a. Solution A—0.2 M $NaH_2PO_4 \cdot H_2O$ 27.6 g/liter

    b. Solution B—0.2 M $Na_2HPO_4 \cdot 7H_2O$ 53.6 g/liter

    c. Washing Buffer—0.005 M PO_4 - 0.3 M NaCl, pH 7.5

         (1) Mix 16 ml Solution A with 84 ml Solution B, dilute to 200 ml, and adjust pH to 7.5.*

         (2) Dilute 25 ml of this buffer to 1 liter to make 0.005 M.

         (3) Dissolve 17.4 g NaCl in 1 liter of the 0.005 M PO_4 buffer to give 0.3 M NaCl.

    d. Eluting Buffer No. 1—pH 8, 0.02 M

         (1) Mix 5.3 ml Solution A with 94.7 ml Solution B, dilute to 200 ml, and adjust pH to 8.*

         (2) Dilute 1/10 for a final molarity of 0.02 M.

    e. Eluting Buffer No. 2—pH 8, 0.3 M

         (1) Mix 5.3 ml $NaH_2PO_4 \cdot H_2O$ (4.1 g/100 ml) with 94.7 ml $Na_2PO_4 \cdot 7H_2O$ (8 g/100 ml), dilute to 200 ml, and adjust pH to 8.*

---

* When making buffers from two stock solutions, 90% of the one to be used in greater volume should be placed in a vessel and balanced to pH by adding the one in lesser volume. In this manner, both molarity and pH are assured. Dilute with an equal amount of distilled water if the full 100 ml of stock solutions have not been used.

2. Preparation of DEAE-Cellulose

a. Suspend 2 g DEAE-cellulose in 1 liter 0.5 M NaCl. Let settle and decant. Repeat this washing procedure three times.

b. Charge the resin by adding 500 ml 0.1 M NaOH and stirring. Let settle and decant.

c. Wash three times with copious amounts of washing buffer and then three times with Eluting Buffer No. 1.

d. Resuspend in fresh buffer, and adjust the pH to 7.5 if necessary after stirring for 15 min.

3. Preparation of Column

a. Use a column at least 30 cm in length and 1 cm I.D.

b. Slowly pour the slurry of buffered resin into the column, and allow the resin to settle evenly. Care should be taken to avoid air bubbles.

c. Begin flowing the initial eluting buffer through the column. The flow rate of buffer through the column should be adjusted from 12 to 15 ml/hr.

d. Prepare a gradient apparatus as follows:

   (1) Suspend a 100-ml beaker on a magnetic stirrer mounted on a ring stand above the column. Connect the beaker to a 50-ml Erlenmeyer flask.

   (2) Place 90 ml Eluting Buffer No. 1 (0.02 M) in the beaker and 55 ml Eluting Buffer No. 2 (0.3 M) in the flask. Connect flask to beaker and beaker to column by siphons. The flow should be from the flask to the beaker to the column.

4. Chromatographing the Sample

a. Stop the flow of the column when the last of the eluting buffer has just entered the column. Do not let the top of the resin column become dry.

b. Carefully layer 10 to 30 mg of protein (serum sample) onto the top of the resin with a capillary pipette. Bending the pipette 180° into a U facilitates sample application with a minimum of resin disturbance.

c. Allow the sample to just enter the resin, stop the flow, and carefully add a small volume of Eluting Buffer No. 1 (0.02 M).

d. Attach a siphon from the gradient mixing chamber (beaker) to the column, and adjust the flow of the column appropriately. The siphon will automatically feed in more buffer as the eluting fluid drops in the column.

e. A total volume of 150 ml of eluant will be sufficient to make a run. Collect samples of eluant in 3- to 4-ml amounts by means of a fraction collector.

f. The samples can be analyzed for protein by optical density at 280 mμ, for immunoglobulin content by immunodiffusion against known antisera, and for antibody activity by appropriate serologic techniques.

2. Rapid Separation of IgM from IgG

The previous technology can assume any form from very precise methods for ultimate resolution to rapid solutions for minor problems. An example of the latter is the availability of small columns prefilled with ion exchange resin and designed for separating two major components. For example, if a 2- to 3-ml column is filled with DEAE-cellulose and attention is paid to the pH or molarity of the wash and elution buffers, one can easily separate IgM from IgG. Since the latter is poorly charged for the resin under conditions of the buffers, most IgG isotypes pass through the column leaving the IgM and certain other globulins behind. These can be eluted separately by passing a different buffer through the column.

It is often important to define which immunoglobulin class specific antibodies are in, such as when it is necessary to know if a newborn infant has been infected *in utero* (antibodies will be IgM) or whether antibodies have passed through the placenta from the mother (IgG). Responses primarily composed of IgM may be indications of early immunization and so on.

If time or equipment is in short supply, it is suggested that this simple experiment be run to demonstrate the principle of ion exchange chromatography.

PROCEDURE

1. This experiment will require the use of commercially available kits (Quik-Sep, Isolab, Inc., Drawer 4350, Akron, OH 44321). The directions that follow pertain to the System II columns, which separate the proteins on the basis of changes in molarity. Buffer nomenclature refers to the two solutions that come with the kit.

2. Prepare a column for use by removing the top cap and then the bottom closure.

3. Allow the fluid above the resin to drain out, and then gently push the separation disc down so that it is just touching the top of the resin bed. Do not compress the resin.

4. Add 2 ml Wash Buffer No. 1 to the column, and drain until the meniscus reaches the top of the disc. This charges the resin. Discard the eluate.

5. Dilute 0.2 ml anti-*Salmonella* serum with 1 ml IgG Wash Buffer, and place the entire amount on the column.

6. Add 4 ml additional IgG Wash Buffer, and let column drain until the meniscus once again reaches the top disc.

7. Collect the eluant, which contains most of the IgG isotypes and will be diluted about 1/26. The IgM will be bound to the column, as will IgG_4.

8. Place a clean test tube under the column, and add 2 ml IgM Elution Buffer.

9. Collect the IgM eluant, which will be diluted 1/10.

10. Assay the eluates for agglutinin activity, and compare with the titer of the original antiserum.

Exercise 14

ELECTROPHORESIS

The motion of a dispersed phase (e.g., colloidal particles) through a dispersion medium (e.g., an electrolyte) under the influence of an electrical potential is known as electrophoresis. This tool has been found to be widely applicable in immunochemistry. The rate of migration of a substance through an electrophoretic field depends on the charge of the particle, pH, voltage of the electric field, composition of the dispersing medium, and length of time of electrophoretic application.

Since proteins are the most frequently involved substances in immunology, we will restrict the discussion to them. Since they are composed of amino acids, all proteins are amphoteric (i.e., they contain radicals that are capable of acting as proton donors and proton acceptors). The relative amounts of these components in a protein determine the sign and the magnitude of the surface charge of the molecule. The charge may be varied by the pH of the dispersing medium. If the charge of the molecule is negative, it will migrate toward the anode in an electrical field. If the charge is reduced to neutrality by adjusting the pH of the medium, the particles will migrate toward neither pole. At this point, the substance is at the isoelectric point. Lowering the pH makes the particles more positively charged, and they migrate toward the cathode.

Since the proteins have different charges, a mixture of them may readily be separated and purified by the process of electrophoresis. When serum is subjected to such a process, albumin is found to migrate fastest towards the anode at pH 8.6, followed by alpha, beta, and gamma globulins in that order. For purposes of this exercise, electrophoretic separation will be carried out in standard veronal buffer (pH 8.6, ionic strength 0.05) by the cellulose acetate technique.

1. Cellulose Acetate Electrophoresis

PROCEDURE

1. Solutions

   a. Buffer—TRIS (Sigma # T 1503)   9.8   g
      Calcium lactate   0.106 g
      Tricine (Sigma # T 0377)   4.3   g
      Distilled water   1000 ml
      Adjust pH to   8.6

   b. Protein stain—Ponceau S   0.4   g
      3% trichloracetic acid   200   ml

   c. Wash solution—5% acetic acid

2. Apparatus

   Any commercial electrophoresis chamber suitable for cellulose acetate strips will suffice. The reservoir generally consists of two pairs of chambers with electrodes being placed in the center member of each pair. The cellulose acetate strips are positioned so that the ends of the strips hang into the outermost member of each pair. The entire reservoir should be enclosed by a transparent cover. Since details may vary with the operation and design of the equipment, consult the manufacturer's instructions for further operating instructions.

3. Technique

   a. Fill the reservoir with an appropriate amount of buffer. Make certain that the buffer is at the same level in each chamber.

   b. Float 2.5-x-13-cm cellulose acetate strips (Gelman Instrument Co., Ann Arbor, MI) on the surface of the buffer solution. Allow the strips to soak at least 30 min.

   c. Carefully blot the strips between sheets of buffer-dampened filter paper, and position them in the electrophoresis chamber.

   d. Apply a 2-μl sample to the strip about one-third of the distance from the cathode. Take care that the line of application across the width of the strip is as straight as possible and that the sample should not be applied closer than 0.5 cm from each margin. This will require practice.

   e. Connect the power supply as soon after application as possible, and adjust to 200 volts. Allow separation to proceed for 90 min.

   f. After the run, float the strips onto the Ponceau S solution, and allow to remain for 5 min.

   g. Transfer the strips to successive washes of 5% acetic acid (3 min each) until the background of each strip is free from stain. Allow to dry and observe results.

2. Immunoelectrophoresis

A finer method of analysis of biological fluids involves the combination of the two techniques of immunodiffusion and electrophoresis. Essentially this technique of immunoelectrophoresis separates the sample components by electrophoresis and subsequently resolves the separated components by immuno-chemical precipitation. The advantage of this technique is that it can resolve multiple components with similar electrophoretic mobilities or antigenically related materials which are electrophoretically hetero-geneous.

Generally, the initial separation is done on an agar gel medium poured onto microscope slides, under conditions similar to those for paper strip electrophoresis. Once the electrophoretic separation is completed, an antiserum is added that contains antibodies known to precipitate the components under investigation. The antiserum is positioned on the slide in such a manner that diffusion will occur perpendicular to the axis of electrophoretic migration. The antibodies precipitate at equivalence with the radially diffusing com-ponents forming arc-shaped lines in the agar. The location of these arcs shows the electrophoretic positions of the antigens, as well as antigenic differences of electrophoretically similar materials.

PROCEDURE

1. Solutions

   a. Buffer—TRIS (Sigma # T 1503)   9.8   g
      Calcium lactate   0.106 g
      Tricine (Sigma # T 0377)   4.3   g
      Distilled water   1000 ml
      Adjust pH to   8.6

b. Immunoelectrophoresis Agar

Purified agar	1	g
Buffer	25	ml
Distilled water	75	ml

c. Impregnation Agar

Agar	0.1	g
Glycerol	0.05	ml
Distilled Water	100	ml

d. Stains and Wash Solutions
1% glycerol
Cold saline
0.1% thiazine red R in 1% acetic acid
70% ethanol containing 1% acetic acid

2. Apparatus

Most paper or cellulose acetate strip electrophoresis outfits are easily adaptable to perform immunoelectrophoresis. Provision should be made for placing the slides in the apparatus in such a fixed position that the electrophoretic run may be made conveniently and safely.

3. Technique

a. Prepare slides by placing alcohol-cleaned and dried slides in hot, melted impregnation agar. Drain and allow to dry in an upright position leaning against a test tube rack overnight.

b. Place the dried, coated slides on a level surface, and pour 2 ml hot immunoelectrophoresis agar on the slide taking care to cover the slide completely. Allow to gel for 2 hr in the cold. The slides should be placed in a moist chamber during this period.

c. Cut suitable patterns in the slides with the device supplied by the manufacturer. Although the details of these devices vary, all of them provide for cutting one or two long narrow troughs and one or two small wells. The agar should be removed from the wells only.

d. Carefully fill the wells with the samples to be analyzed, and place the slides in the apparatus.

e. Gently attach buffer-dampened filter paper wicks 1″ x 2.5″ to each end of each slide and allow the free end of each wick to hang in the buffer. When finished, each slide and wick combination should complete a circuit by bridging the two chambers.

f. Connect the power supply, and adjust to 150 V. Allow to proceed for 90 min.

g. Turn off the power supply at the end of the run, remove the slides from the apparatus, discarding the wicks, and carefully remove the agar from the troughs.

h. Charge the troughs with the appropriate precipitating antiserum, and replace the slides in the moist chamber. Incubate the slides for 48 hr at 4°C.

i. After incubation, observe and record the precipitation patterns.

j. The slides may be stained and preserved at this point if desired. First wash the slides at 4°C for 36 hr with copious amounts of cold saline. Each slide should be placed in a separate 250-ml beaker for this.

k. Place in 1% glycerol for 15 min, drain, and air dry for 3 to 5 hr in a low-temperature (40°C) drying oven.

l. Stain with the thiazine red R solution for 60 min.

m. Clarify specific staining by removing background stain with 70% ethanol and 1% glycerol for 15 min.

n. Rinse in distilled water for 30 min and 1% glycerol for 15 min.

o. Re-air dry. The stained slides may then be kept indefinitely.

Suggested Uses of Immunoelectrophoresis

1. Electrophorese normal human serum (undiluted and 1/5 dilutions on same slide) and develop with commercial *goat* anti-human serum.

2. Compare with serum from a patient with multiple myeloma (often commercially available).

3. Electrophorese fractions from gel filtration or chromatography experiments, and develop with appropriate goat antisera.

4. Electrophorese fresh *human* serum activated with inulin, and develop with anti-human C3PA (Factor B).

Exercise 15
IMMUNOHISTOCHEMISTRY

The combination of the precision of histochemical staining with the specificity of serological reactions has resulted in a powerful tool in the study of tissues and other microscopic forms. In such procedures, purified antibodies are either chemically or serologically attached to a chemical marker that is easily seen microscopically. When such materials are used as stains, specific antigen becomes tagged visually. The widespread use of the technique of immunofluorescence involves the chemical coupling of antibody globulin to dyes capable of emitting visible fluorescence when excited with ultraviolet light. A newer method involves the building of a serological bridge between the specific antibody and the enzyme peroxidase. The section with the bound peroxidase is then developed chemically with an appropriate substrate that then becomes visible microscopically.

1. Immunofluorescence

Certain fluorescent dyes such as the isocyanate derivatives of fluorescein and rhodamine and the dye lissamine rhodamine B are easily conjugated with proteins. Isocyanates freely associate with terminal amino groups of protein chains and possibly with free sulfhydryl groups. Thus, since these reactions are nonspecific, it is important that extraneous protein be removed and that the antibody preparation be of the highest purity. When using a properly prepared conjugate, a tissue culture slide or impression smear is allowed to react or "stain" with the specific antibody labeled with fluorescein isothiocyanate. After an appropriate washing, the smear may be viewed through a UV microscope. If there were antigen present in the smear and if an appropriate specific globulin were used, an antigen-antibody reaction would be evidenced by the retention of fluorescent staining in those areas containing antigen.

When the specific antiserum is conjugated and used as stain in the procedure, it is termed *direct immunofluorescence*. This differs from *indirect immunofluorescence* is that with the latter the slide is stained with labeled antiglobulin. Ths results are the same, but the latter is considered more sensitive and only one labeling procedure is required instead of several, one for each antiserum.

For students unfamiliar with these techniques, a warning must be given. The results are not as easy to achieve as the above indicates due to nonspecific staining of various types. First of all, most tissues have some degree of blue-white autofluorescence, but this is easily distinguished from the apple green color of fluorescein isothiocyanate. However, the intensity of the autofluorescence may mask specific fluorescence. Secondly, certain tissues nonspecifically stain with fluorescein isothiocyanate alone (e.g., certain parts of leukocytes, the internal elastic membranes of the larger veins and bronchioles, and the stratum corneum of the epidermis composed of keratin). A third type of nonspecific staining is due to unexplained impurities of the dye and/or the globulin. This can be alleviated to some degree by using purified crystalline dye and purer globulins such as might be obtained by column chromatography. A fourth type of staining is due to cross reactivity of the globulin preparation with heterologous antigens, which of course can be remedied by specific cross adsorption. For instance, antisera prepared by immunizing animals with cell culture supernates should be adsorbed with cells of that culture system. Antigenic materials such as serum used as enrichment in all culture systems should obviously be avoided if possible. A true interpretation of immunofluorescence necessitates the strictest attention to detail and the use of rigid controls.

PROCEDURE

1. Solutions

   a. 0.85% NaCl

   b. Carbonate-bicarbonate buffer

Solution A	Na_2CO_3	5.3 g
	Distilled water	100 ml
Solution B	$NaHCO_3$	4.2 g
	Distilled water	100 ml

   Fresh solutions should be prepared as needed. Add 4.4 ml solution A to 100 ml solution B. The final pH should be 9.0.

   c. Phosphate-buffered saline

Solution A	Na_2HPO_4	1.4 g
	Distilled water	100 ml
Solution B	$NaH_2PO_4H_2O$	1.4 g
	Distilled water	100 ml

   Add 84.1 ml solution A to 15.9 ml solution B. Add 8.5 g NaCl, and dilute to 1 liter with distilled water. The final pH should be 7.6.

   d. 0.1% fluorescein isothiocyanate in carbonate-bicarbonate buffer.

2. Precipitation and Conjugation of Immune Globulins

   a. Precipitate the globulin in 5 ml of an antibacterial serum* (see EXERCISE 12). Desalt the dissolved precipitate accordingly.

   b. Perform a biuret determination on the desalted globulin solution. Multiply the volume in milliliters of solution times the number of milligrams protein/milliliter to give the total amount of protein.

   c. Calculate how much solvent must be added to the globulin solution to effect a 1% or 10 mg/ml concentration. Next, multiply the total protein times 0.02 to give the amount of crystalline dye necessary for conjugation.

   Example:
   (1) 2.7 ml globulin after gel filtration at 18 mg/ml = 48.6 mg
   2.7 ml x 18 mg = V ml x 10 mg
   V = 4.86 ml final volume of protein

   (2) 48.6 mg protein x 0.02 = 0.972 mg dye necessary

   Therefore add 0.97 ml dye solution to the 2.7 ml globulin, which will give you a total of 3.67 ml.

   (3) But you need a total volume of 4.86 ml or approximately 1.2 ml more diluent to bring the final concentration of protein up to 10 mg/ml. Add this amount of carbonate-bicarbonate buffer to the solution.

   d. Incubate this mixture in an ice bath for at least 6 hr. At the end of this time, the unconjugated dye must be removed by dialysis against phosphate-buffered saline in the cold

---

* Suggested systems: Streptococci (Group A), *Salmonella,* etc., with the appropriate antiserum.

for 48 hr or passed through a G-25 Sephadex column equilibrated with phosphate-buffered saline.*

    e.   This material may be assayed for antibody titer, used immediately, stored frozen, or lyophilized.

3. Staining

    a.   After drying the smears of the appropriate organisms, fix in 95% ethanol for 1 min, drain, dip in PBS, and dry.

    b.   It may be necessary to determine beforehand the optimum dilution of conjugate to use in staining as prozones do occur in FA work. Cover the area on one slide (A) with conjugate, another slide (B) with normal globulin conjugate, and a third slide (C) with unconjugated antiserum. Place all slides in a moist chamber for 30 to 60 min.

    c.   Wash all slides in three changes of phosphate-buffered saline and one final change of distilled water for 5 min each.

    d.   Mount slides A and B in buffered glycerol (9 parts glycerin/1 part phosphate buffer). Stain slide C with specific conjugate, rewash as in step C, and mount in buffered glycerol.

4. UV Microscopy

    a.   Center the condenser under a low-powered objective with dark field illumination.

    b.   Using an ultraviolet absorbing glass eyepiece filter and either a 2-, 3-, or 5-mm UV transmission filter, observe the section under ultraviolet light at medium power for the specific apple green fluorescence. This specific fluorescence should be seen in the cells from slide A. No such staining should be seen in the cells on slides B and C. Cover slip C is a check for the specificity of the stain.

    c.   If time does not permit making one's own conjugates, fluorescein labeled antirabbit globulin may be purchased commercially, and the indirect method can be applied to this same system. Outline a protocol including controls for carrying out this procedure before proceeding.

    d.   It will be necessary to know or to determine the titer of anti-globulin conjugates whether commercially obtained or self-made. Titers are obtained by means of gel diffusion tests carried out on agar-coated microscope slides. Serial dilutions of anti-globulin are placed in 2.8-mm peripheral wells arranged 7.5 mm from a central well containing the globulin at a 1-mg/ml concentration. The titer is the highest dilution of antiserum giving a line of reaction against the antigen. The titer is the unitage (i.e., a 1/8 titer = 8 units/ml). The use dilution of conjugated anti-globulin is usually at this dilution.

Suggested Experiments for Immunofluorescence

1. Fixed smears of *E. coli* or *S. typhi* and antiserum produced from EXERCISE 2.

2. Frozen kidney sections from rats in EXERCISE 17 stained from fluorescent labeled antirabbit globulin.

3. Fixed impression smears of spleen sections from mice injected four days previously with antigen and stained with labeled anti-mouse globulin.

4. Fixed smears of human buffy coat stained with labeled anti-human globulin (identifies B lymphocytes). Interpret data in light of EXERCISE 5.

---

* NOTE: Sephadex will not be reusable once it has been stained with dye.

Section IV

IMMUNOPATHOLOGY

The immune response must always be considered a two-edged sword in that not only can the system neutralize noxious agents and defend the body from foreign or mutational insult, but it can also result in damage to the host as a consequence of a primary antigen-antibody reaction. This section will examine the four major ways such immune injury may be brought about.

Reagin or IgE dependent. Special classes of antibody have the ability to fix via their Fc fractions to basophiles, mast cells, and certain other specialized cells. When these antibodies react with antigen through the Fab end of the molecules, a stress is transmitted to the affixed cells, causing them to release various pharmocologically active substances that bring about the manifestations of immediate hypersensitivities.

Cytotoxicity. Cytotoxicity results when the antigen is either a part of the cell or has become attached to the cell. Subsequent reaction with antibody results in damage or death to that cell. Often these reactions are accompanied by complement fixation, which activates other tissue-damaging mechanisms.

Immune complex. Soluble antigen-antibody complexes fix complement and attract neutrophiles to the site of deposit of the complexes. The lysosomal enzymes released by these cells bring about the tissue damage.

Cell mediated. Unlike the first three, these reactions are cell dependent and result in the delayed type of hypersensitivity. Specifically sensitized lymphocytes react with antigen causing the release of lymphokines or soluble, macromolecular mediators that bring about various forms of tissue damage.

Due to the special nature of these experiments, many are not suitable as classroom experiments, but are perhaps better carried out as demonstrations, special projects, or group experiments. Many of the animals must be pre-immunized so it is recommended that a master schedule be set up ahead of time indicating what has to be done on what day. In this way, the instructor may have available his or her precise needs at the times desired. One proven method is to assign a group the preparation of the contact sensitivity, an individual the Arthus rabbit, and so on, specifying the dates necessary to have the indicated animals ready for demonstration.

Exercise 16

IMMEDIATE HYPERSENSITIVITY

Immediate hypersensitivity is characterized by initial contact with an antigen, the production of circulating antibody, the ability to be passively transferred by serum, and the effect on vascular tissue and smooth muscle after a reaction. In most forms of immediate hypersensitivity, the presence of histamine and/or certain other substances following the reactions can be demonstrated. These substances alone have the ability to produce strikingly similar reactions when injected into normal control animals.

Perhaps the best-known type of immediate hypersensitivity is anaphylaxis. If animals such as humans, dogs, or guinea pigs are sensitized with certain antigens and later contact this antigen in adequate amounts, an extremely severe pathologic syndrome results.

The best animal for the demonstration of anaphylaxis is the guinea pig sensitized with an antigen such as egg albumin or horse serum. The condition is also dependent on the route and amount of the sensitizing and shocking doses and the interval between these doses. If the animal survives anaphylaxis, it will be temporarily refractory to more shocking doses. However, after a suitable rest for two to three days, the animal will be as sensitive, if not more so, as it was before.

1. Anaphylaxis

PROCEDURE

1. Sensitize pairs of 400- to 600-g guinea pigs by each of the following methods:

    a. Active—0.1 ml horse serum I. P. 19 days before shock
       0.1 ml horse serum I. P. 17 days before shock
       0.1 ml horse serum I. P. 15 days before shock

    b. Active—0.1 ml horse serum diluted 1/100 I. P. 10 to 11 days before shock

    c. Passive—1 ml high-titered anti-horse serum intracardially 6 to 24 hr prior to shock dose

2. The shocking dose for each animal at the specified time is performed by injecting 2 to 3 ml horse serum intracardially.

3. Observe and record the symptoms of each animal after shocking. Autopsy any animals that die, noting especially the inflated character of the lungs and the presence of minute hemorrhages.

4. Reshock any animals that have recovered 30 to 60 min after recovery. Explain the results. If time permits, reshock these animals 1 week later and observe.

    NOTE: Some instructors may wish to videotape a good demonstration of this experiment so that animals need not be killed each time of demonstration.

2. Passive Cutaneous Anaphylaxis

Advantage may be taken of the immediate hypersensitivity phenomenon to develop a sensitive method for the demonstration of an antigen-antibody reaction. In this procedure, skin sites of a guinea pig are passively sensitized with a suitable antibody. After allowing a sufficient time to elapse for the fixation of the antibody to these tissues, the animal is challenged with a mixture of the antigen and suitable dye given intravenously. The reaction that takes place causes a rapid accumulation of dye in the subepidermal tissues surrounding the sensitized skin site as a result of dilatation of the venules and capillaries. These vessels become damaged and permeable to plasma fluids and hence the dye becomes manifest by leaking into these areas. This procedure does not detect human IgE, but will if subhuman primates are used as the test animals.

PROCEDURE

1. Depilate the flanks and abdomen of each of several 300- to 400-g guinea pigs.

2. Inject intradermally 0.1-ml dilutions of sterile anti-bovine serum albumin into separate sites, beginning with a 1/20 dilution. Include a saline control.

3. After 6 hr, slowly inject 0.2 ml 5% bovine serum albumin together with 1 ml of a 1% Evans blue solution intracardially (0.25 ml/100 g body weight).

4. Make observations at the end of 30 min and 60 min, respectively. An area of dye infiltration must measure at least 7 mm in diameter. Some observers prefer to sacrifice the animal at the end of 50 min and reflect the skin in order to observe the reaction, but this is unnecessary.

3. Action of Histamine and Antihistamines

Many of the symptoms of the immediate type of hypersensitivity are thought to be due to histamine which seems to be released from tissue as a side reaction to the antigen-antibody combinations. Indeed, histamine injected into a normal animal alone will produce many anaphylactic-type symptoms. This has led to the use of antihistaminic drugs (not antibodies, but competitive inhibitors) in the prevention or alleviation of allergic symptoms.

PROCEDURE

1. Inject guinea pigs intracardially with 0.25 mg histamine. Observe results, and perform autopsies as before.

2. Inject other guinea pigs (previously sensitized with horse serum) intraperitoneally with 6 to 10 mg Benadryl (Parke, Davis and Co., Detroit, MI).

3. Thirty minutes after administration of the antihistamine, shock the animal with antigen by the method described above. Compare the results with those of unprotected guinea pigs.

Exercise 17
CYTOTOXIC REACTIONS

When humoral antibody reacts with a cellular antigen, often also involving the fixation of complement, the result may be toxic for the cell. These reactions may be subclassified into several types. In one type of reaction, the antigen is an intrinsic or integral part of the cell as in the case of the glomerular basement membrane antigen involved in one form of immunologic glomerulonephritis. If the individual produces antibody against antigens of this nature, the process of autoimmunity results and is often destructive.

A second form of reaction involves extrinsic antigens being adsorbed to host cells in such a way that when subsequent reaction with antibody takes place, damage to the cell results. Such a process is known to take place in the disease idiopathic thrombocytopenic purpura, in which antibodies reacting with certain drugs having a nonspecific attachment to platelets cause a decrease in the number of platelets, resulting in an impairment to the clotting mechanism.

A third type of cytotoxic reaction occurs when extrinsic antigens have the same specificity as antigens found in host tissue. One of the most studied examples of this type is the streptococcal cell membrane antigen that shares a coincidental specificity with a myofibrillar antigen of heart muscle. It is believed that the cardiac lesions of rheumatic fever are due to streptococcal antibodies cross-reacting with the cardiac antigens.

PROCEDURE

A. Masugi Nephritis—Although strictly a heteroimmune phenomenon, this simplified procedure will illustrate the principles and techniques of autoimmunity.

1. Homogenize the kidneys of ten healthy rats in phosphate-buffered saline with a suitable tissue homogenizer to effect a 20% suspension.

2. Prepare two antigen-Freund's adjuvant mixtures, one complete and one incomplete (see EXERCISE 2) from this suspension.

3. Immunize rabbits according to the following schedule:

   First day—1 ml Freund's complete-antigen I. P.
   Fifth day—1 ml Freund's incomplete-antigen I. D.
   Continue I. P. injections with the incomplete adjuvant-antigen mixture every four days for two more weeks. Allow animals to rest one week before bleeding and harvesting serum.

4. In order to produce glomerulonephritis, inject rats intravenously with 0.5 ml/100 g body weight of the nephrotoxic serum. Inoculate the rats every four days for a total of six injections.

5. One week after the final injection, sacrifice the animals including a control, remove the kidneys, and prepare for frozen sectioning.

6. Fix the frozen sections in 50-50 ethanol ether for 10 min at room temperature followed by 20 min in 95% ethanol at 37°C.

7. The sections are then given two 5-min phosphate-buffered saline washes before staining. Drain sections, but do not blot.

8. Stain the sections with 1/20 anti-rabbit globulin conjugated with fluorescein isothiocyanate for 30 min.

9. Give sections two 5-min PBS washes, one 5-min distilled water wash, and mount in buffered glycerol.

10. Examine mounted sections with the UV microscope and observe the brilliant fluorescence of the glomeruli. Compare with the control. If available, stain additional sections by a conventional hematoxylin and eosin method and observe the cortical necrosis, cellular infiltration, and tubular edema.

Exercise 18

IMMUNE COMPLEX REACTIONS

Immune complex reactions are due to precipitating antibodies reacting with extrinsic antigen in regions of antigen excess resulting in soluble antigen-antibody complexes. Such complexes fix complement, attract neutrophiles, and cause platelet aggregation, all of which lead to tissue injury. Such a mechanism is responsible for the dermal Arthus reaction, part of the serum sickness syndrome, the most common immunologic form of glomerulonephritis, allergic vasculitis, and certain other pathologic manifestations. These manifestations are due to the site of localization of the complexes, which in turn affect the deposition of the hydrolytic enzymes released by the neutrophiles attracted to the complexes.

This exercise will examine two of the classic forms of immune complex reactions *in vivo*.

1. The Arthus Reaction

The Arthus phenomenon is due to antigen-antibody reactions that cause pathology. The tissue reaction is characterized by edema and necrosis at the site of antigen injection. The mechanism is thought to be due to a direct result of antigen-antibody precipitates being formed within the vascular tissues. The antibody must be present in high titer and must be of the precipitating type. Histamine and similar substances are not released by this mechanism; hence antihistamines are ineffectual in preventing or ameliorating the reaction.

PROCEDURE

1. Inject 0.1 ml 1% ovalbumin solution intradermally into a rabbit once every three days.

2. Continue injections until an immediate reaction takes place at the site of the last injection. Succeeding injections should yield even more accentuated reactions. It may take as many as 11 to 12 such injections before a suitable reaction level is obtained.

2. Glomerulonephritis

Perhaps the best studied immunopathologic reaction is immune complex-induced glomerulonephritis. This is produced in animals immunized to foreign antigens who respond by producing precipitins in the presence of excessive amounts of free antigen. This results in the production of circulating, soluble antigen-antibody complexes. If this continues, these complexes are deposited on the glomerular basement membranes of the kidney, where they fix complement and attract neutrophils. The latter release their lysosomal enzymes, causing damage to the membranes. The gaps formed in the membranes allow the immune deposits to move through to the epithelial side of the membranes. If stained with fluorescent-labeled antiglobulin, the glomeruli reveal the presence of discrete, "lumpy-dumpy" deposits, thus distinguishing them from the type examined in the preceding exercise. If the complexes are large enough to precipitate out, they are phagocytized before localizing; if they are found in large excesses of antigen, they do not seem to localize in the glomeruli as well; hence the ratio of antigen to antibody in the complexes seems to be quite critical for the production of this pathology.

PROCEDURE

1. It is suggested that this extended experiment be conducted as a class project, thereby dividing up the injections. It will be necessary to hyperimmunize rabbits over a period of several weeks with daily intravenous injections of antigens. Because not every animal produces the disease, it is recommended to immunize more than one rabbit.

2. Begin by injecting I. V. each rabbit with 10 mg per rabbit each day five to six days per week with bovine or human serum albumin.

3. During the second week of immunization, bleed the rabbits and do equivalent proportion titrations on the sera. On animals producing large amounts of antibody, change the daily dose of antigen to 30 or 50 mg daily. Rebleed the animals to see if the level of antibody has been partially neutralized. Try to balance the daily dose of antigen with the amount of antibody produced so that the animals are near equivalence. Discard any animals not responding by the third week.

4. After five to six weeks of such treatment, sacrifice the animal and remove the kidneys. Prepare frozen sections and fix in 95% alcohol at 37° C for 15 min.

5. Rehydrate in FA-PBS (see p. 87) for 5 min and then proceed to stain with specific immuno-chemical conjugates (e.g., anti-BSA or HSA, anti-rabbit globulin, and anti-complement). Proceed according to directions under EXERCISE 15, Immunofluorescence.

6. Observe for focal, granular patterns of immunofluorescence in glomeruli by means of ultraviolet microscopy.

Exercise 19

CELL-MEDIATED REACTIONS

Unlike the preceding reactions that have all been due to various forms of humoral antibody, these reactions are due to cell-mediated immunity or delayed-type hypersensitivity. The classic example of this type is the delayed skin reaction to tuberculin seen in tuberculosis sensitization. Such a reaction plays a significant role in the pathogenesis of lesion formation in cavitary tuberculosis and in certain other infectious diseases.

The principal cells responsible for this type of reaction are the thymus-dependent lymphocytes. When specifically sensitized lymphocytes react with antigen, a variety of effector macromolecules known as lymphokines are released that account for such manifestations as migration inhibition of macrophages, target-cell cytotoxicity, mitogenesis, chemotaxis, and transfer of specific sensitivity. These features combine in an intricately interwoven sequence of events *in vivo* that result in the gross and histological appearance of the lesion. The cell-mediated type of immunity is responsible for protection against many viral and bacterial pathogens, graft rejection, and probably most importantly, the day-to-day homeostatic policing of the body from the development of mutant or neoplastic cells.

1. Delayed Hypersensitivity

Delayed hypersensitivity includes allergy of infection and contact allergy and differs from the immediate type in that it requires prolonged initial contact, no circulating antibody can be demonstrated, and that the reaction, as the name indicates, is classically delayed 48 to 72 hr after secondary contact. Also, there does not seem to be any specific shock organ involved as in the immediate type, and passive transfer has been adequately demonstrated with leukocytic transfer only. Delayed hypersensitivity is responsible for much of the host-parasite interaction in such chronic diseases as tuberculosis.

PROCEDURE

    A.   Allergy to Infection

        1.   Sensitize guinea pigs by injecting 0.5 ml Freund's complete adjuvant (made with killed TB bacilli, not *Mycobacterium butyricum*) intramuscularly into each hind leg three weeks prior to testing.

        2.   Depilate a 4-in square of skin on the flank of the animal.

        3.   Inject 0.1 ml PPD (Second Strength) intradermally into the depilated area.

        4.   Observe the reaction at the end of 48 hr and 72 hr. Note any changes that have occurred in this period.

    B.   Contact Dermatitis

        1.   Depilate the skin from a 2-in square on the flank of six to eight guinea pigs. Allow 24 hr to elapse before further treatment.

2. Divide the animals into two groups. Using a glass stirring rod, stroke 0.2 to 0.3 ml absolute ethanol into the skin of each animal in the control group. Repeat daily applications for a total of seven days.

3. Repeat this procedure with the animals in the test group, using a 2% solution of 2,4-dinitro-chlorobenzene (DNCB) in absolute ethanol.

4. After three weeks, again depilate the animals at the treated sites, and allow any inflammation to subside for 24 hr.

5. Into separate 1-cm^2 areas of each animal, stroke 0.1-ml samples of 0.25% and 0.1% solutions of DNCB in absolute ethanol, respectively.

6. Make observations at 24-hr and 48-hr intervals on both groups of guinea pigs.

2. Migration Inhibition Factor (MIF)

The discovery and development of methods for the demonstration of *in vitro* correlates of delayed hypersensitivity have revolutionized the study of cellular immunity and placed it on a much firmer scientific foundation. One of the first such factors studied was the production of a substance from antigen-lymphocyte culture supernates that inhibited the normal migration of macrophages. Several methods have been devised for demonstrating this factor, MIF, and currently its production is considered to result from antigen-specific stimulation and to be a good, but not absolute, *in vitro* correlate of the delayed hypersensitivity skin reaction.

PROCEDURE

A. Sensitized Cell Preparation

1. Inject 20 to 25 ml sterile mineral oil I. P. in a guinea pig previously immunized with BCG in a manner similar to that of the preceding experiment. (It is suggested that another student [or group] proceed similarly with an unimmunized animal.)

2. After five days, sacrifice the animal by anesthesia and, using aseptic technique, reflect the abdominal skin.

3. About midway between the groin and diaphragm, cut a 4- to 5-cm slit in the muscular wall into the peritoneal cavity.

4. At each end of the slit place a hemostat, and suspend from a ring stand in such a way as to raise the muscle wall to produce a well in the cavity.

5. Aseptically pour 120 ml Hanks balanced salt solution (HBSS) into the cavity, and knead gently, taking care not to rupture any vessels or intestines.

6. Withdraw exudate by pipetting the fluid through the perforated plastic tube. The yield should be approximately 120 ml.

7. Centrifuge the suspension at 500 x g for 10 min.

8. Carefully draw off mineral oil and supernates. Discard.

9. Pool cells in small centrifuge tube, and wash 3X in heparinized HBSS at 500 x g.

10. After the last wash, resuspend in Hanks Minimal Essential Medium (MEM) with 15% normal guinea pig serum by adding 1 ml medium for each 0.1 ml packed cells.

B. Assay

1. You will need one chamber for each antigen and one chamber as the reference.

2. Fill capillary tubes with cell suspensions from the sensitized animal. Fill additional tubes with cells from the control.

3. Seal the capillary tubes with sterile clay, and centrifuge at 1300 rpm in a hematocrit centrifuge for $1^1/2$ min (the cells should be spun only enough to pull them to the bottom without packing them tightly).

4. Score the tubes just at the cell-liquid interface, rotate the tube 180°, and break. This should give a clean, even break in the tube.

5. Place one tube from each animal in the chamber so that the sealed ends are facing the ports and held in place by the silicone grease.

6. To one chamber, add 5 to 15 µg PPD. Do not add antigen to the reference chamber. If a third chamber is available, place 30 µg heterologous protein antigen in it. Seal with cover slips and paraffin.

7. Gently fill the chamber with MEM containing 15% normal guinea pig serum, using a syringe fitted with a 27-gauge needle.

8. Seal the access ports with paraffin, and incubate horizontally at 37°C for 24 to 48 hr. (It is helpful to rest the assembled chamber on two applicator sticks in a Petri dish. This assures that any warped chamber may remain level.)

9. After incubation, project the areas of cellular migration, using a viewing screen attachment for the microscope and a 3.5X objective lens.

10. Trace the area of migration, and measure by planimeter if available. (If a planimeter is unavailable, cut out the tracings, and weigh each.)

Calculate:

$$\text{Migration index } = \frac{\text{Area of migration with Ag}}{\text{Area of migration without Ag}} \text{ X } 100$$

An inhibition of greater than 30% (MI = 70 or less) is regarded as significant.

11. Additional points to keep in mind:

a. Do not centrifuge harder than what is described.

b. Maintain pH of all media between 7.2 to 7.4. If adjustment is necessary, do so with sodium bicarbonate or gaseous CO_2, not acid or base.

c. Work should progress as quickly as possible from time of cell harvest to incubation of chamber.

d. All reagents should be kept cold to ensure greatest cellular viability.

e. For greatest reproduction, keep cellular concentrations as close as possible.

3. Autoimmunity—Allergic Encephalomyelitis

Although some forms of autoimmunity involve humoral antibody (EXERCISE 17), the main form of tissue destruction in this kind of disease appears to be cell mediated. Many of these diseases are experimentally induced but are believed to be counterparts of certain spontaneous diseases of humans. This experiment deals with one of the most classic experimental autoimmune diseases, allergic encephalomyelitis.

PROCEDURE

1. Aseptically harvest the brain and spinal cord of a guinea pig. To remove the spinal cord, sever the spinal column at the base of the skull and at the base of the tail. Place a short 20-gauge needle into the exposed canal at the tail, attach a syringe, and carefully force air into the spinal column. The cord should be ejected from the anterior end.

2. Add enough sterile phosphate-buffered saline to make a 1/3 suspension, and homogenize in a sterile blender.

3. Prepare a complete Freund's adjuvant-antigen mixture from this suspension. Save some of the suspension for skin testing.

4. Inject 0.1 ml brain-adjuvant mixture into a foot pad of each hind leg of each guinea pig. Immunize at least three animals.

5. After 10 to 12 days, skin test the guinea pigs with brain suspension (0.1 ml), and observe for delayed hypersensitivity reactions. Neurological symptoms should begin 14 to 21 days after immunization.

Appendix

LABORATORY SUPPLIES

NOTE: In addition to the supplies listed below for each experiment, the laboratory should also have adequate water baths, microscopes, centrifuges, assorted serological pipettes, and microtiter equipment.

EXERCISE 1: Manipulation of Serological Glassware

1. Titration of a Surface Active Agent

   a. 1 ml 0.1% saponin in saline per student
   b. 5 ml 2% erythrocyte suspension per student
   c. Ten 12-x-75-mm tubes per student
   d. 5 ml saline per test

2. Titration of a Precipitinogen

   a. Seven small-bore (5-mm I. D.) tubes per student
   b. Seven 12-x-75-mm tubes per student
   c. 3 ml anti-bovine serum per student
   d. 0.2 ml bovine serum per student
   e. 7 ml saline per test

3. Use of Microtiter Equipment

   a. 1 ml saline per student
   b. 50 μl anti-sheep RBC serum diluted 1/10 per student
   c. One plastic microtiter plate per student
   d. 0.25 ml 2% sheep RBC suspension per student
   e. Microtiter pipettes and disposable, yellow tips

EXERCISE 2: Preparation of Immunizing Agents

1. Bacterial Vaccines

   a. Two 8-oz prescription bottles per student containing 20 ml Trypticase soy agar that has been allowed to solidify with the bottle laying on its side
   b. One 24-hr Trypticase soy broth culture of a flagellated *Salmonella* species per pair of students
   c. Two 20-ml screw-cap test tubes per student
   d. Sterile formal-saline (0.6% formalin in saline)—approximately 2 to 3 liters per class of 12
   e. Absolute ethanol
   f. Sterile cotton-stoppered pipettes
   g. Sets of McFarland's nephelometer tubes
   h. Two 30-ml sterile vaccine vials per student
   i. Two tubes thioglycollate broth per student

2. Viral Vaccines

   a. Two 11-day-old embryonated eggs per student
   b. Influenza virus type A diluted in saline 10^{-1}
   c. Two sterile 10-ml syringes and 20-gauge needles per student
   d. Two 10- to 15-ml sterile centrifuge tubes per student
   e. Class stock of 37% formaldehyde

3. Erythrocyte Antigens

   a. 10 ml sterile citrated blood
   b. Sterile 12-ml centrifuge tubes
   c. Sterile 30-ml vaccine vials
   d. Sterile saline
   e. Sterile pipettes

4. Protein Solutions

    a. Sterile centrifuge tubes
    b. Sterile 15-ml vaccine vials
    c. Aqueous Merthiolate 1/1000 (Eli Lilly and Co., Indianapolis, IN)
    d. Bacteriological filtering apparatus

5. Adjuvants

    a. 2 to 5 ml antigen per preparation
    b. One 5-ml syringe with a 20-gauge needle
    c. Vials of Freund's complete and incomplete adjuvant (Difco Laboratories, Detroit, MI)
    d. 10% aluminum potassium sulfate

EXERCISE 3: Innate Immunity

1. Bactericidal Power of Normal Serum

    a. 1.5 ml fresh normal unheated rabbit serum per pair
    b. 1.5 ml normal heated (56°C/30 min) rabbit serum per pair
    c. Three 9-ml sterile saline blanks per pair
    d. Two 9.9-ml sterile saline blanks per pair
    e. Nine 10-ml melted Trypticase soy agar deeps per pair
    f. Nine sterile Petri dishes per pair
    g. Nine sterile cotton-stoppered test tubes (12-x-75-mm) per pair
    h. Sterile cotton-stoppered pipettes
    i. 24-hr Trypticase soy broth cultures of *Salmonella* species
    j. 24-hr Trypticase soy broth cultures of *Staphylococcus aureus*

2. Clearance of Blood by the Reticuloendothelial System

    a. One 5- to 6-lb rabbit
    b. One 24-hr nutrient agar slant culture of *Escherichia coli*. Emulsify growth in 5 ml sterile saline, and inject 1 ml I. V. of this in experiment
    c. One sterile needle and syringe for injection
    d. Three sterile needles and syringes for bleeding
    e. Sterile pipettes
    f. Three sterile mortars and pestles or Waring blenders
    g. Three 100-ml portions of sterile saline
    h. Three 9-ml sterile saline blanks per student
    i. Three 9.9-ml sterile saline blanks per student
    j. Three 10-ml melted nutrient agar tubes per student
    k. Three sterile Petri dishes per student

3. Phagocytosis Leukocyte Differential Counts

    a. Leukocyte Differential Counts
        (1) Sterile lancets, cotton pledgets, 70% alcohol, and microscope slides
        (2) Wright's stain and methanol

    b. Demonstration of Phagocytosis *in Vivo*
        (1) Six mice per lab
        (2) 24-hr broth culture of *Staphylococcus aureus*
        (3) Sterile 1-ml syringes and 27-gauge needles
        (4) Autopsy instruments and chloroform
        (5) Wright's stain, methanol, and microscope slides

4. Phagocytic Dysfunction

   These are the materials necessary for one group of four students:

   a. 18-hr Trypticase soy culture of *Staphlococcus aureus*
   b. 18 ml filter-sterilized 6% dextran (M.W. 100,000-200,000) containing 50 units heparin/ml
   c. Sterile heparinized saline (25 units/100 ml)
   d. 8 ml Hanks balanced salt solution (Flow Laboratories, Inc., Rockville, MD)
   e. 4 mg hydrocortisone-21-succinate (Sigma Chemical Co., St. Louis, MO)
   f. 1000 units heparin
   g. Sterile 12-ml syringe and 18-gauge needle
   h. Eight sterile screw-cap centrifuge tubes
   i. Six sterile Petri dishes
   j. Two sterile glass test tubes with caps
   k. Sterile capillary pipettes
   l. Sterile cotton plugged pipettes
   m. Six tubes of nutrient agar, melted
   n. Seven 9-ml sterile water blanks
   o. One 9.9-ml sterile water blank

5. Nitroblue Tetrazolium (NBT) Reduction Assay

   a. Trypticase soy culture of *Staphylococcus aureus* (18-hr culture, washed twice, and resuspended in 10 ml saline)
   b. 0.5 ml blood, drawn in heparin per student
   c. 10 ml 0.2% nitroblue tetrazolium (NBT) (Sigma Chemical Co., St. Louis, MO) in preweighed vials (Cat. No. 840-10) or in a kit containing all necessary reagents for assay (Cat. No. 840-A)
   d. Two 12-x-75-mm test tubes per student
   e. Two microscope slides per student
   f. Wright's stain

6. Superoxide Anion Production

   a. 10 ml 6% dextran (M.W. 100,000-200,000) (Sigma) in saline
   b. 500 ml Hanks balanced salt solution (HBSS) (GIBCO, Grand Island, NY)
   c. Opsonized zymosan. Suspend washed zymosan particles, 3 to 5 μ (Nutritional Biochemicals Corp., Chagrin Falls, OH) in saline, and boil for 1 min. Wash boiled particles twice with saline, and resuspend in HBSS containing 10% normal human serum to a concentration of 20 mg/ml
   d. 3 ml cytochrome C, Type III (Sigma, C 2506) solution 15 mg/ml in HBSS
   e. 17-x-100-mm plastic culture tubes
   f. Disposable cellulose acetate filters, 0.45 μ (that attach to a syringe)

EXERCISE 4: Immunoglobulins

1. Ultracentrifugation of Macroglobulins

   This experiment requires a preliminary demonstration of the use of an ultracentrifuge with a swinging bucket rotor. These are the materials necessary for a small group of students:

   a. 1 ml serum in which a known, easily detectable macroglobulin is present (The appropriate titer of the unfractionated serum should be known.)
   b. Appropriate antigen
   c. Two cellulose nitrate tubes (Beckman No. 305050, 1/2″ x 2″)

 d. 3.5 ml 37% sucrose solution in PBS
 e. 3.5 ml 25% sucrose solution in PBS
 f. 3.5 ml 10% sucrose solution in PBS
 g. Two 26-gauge needles
 h. 2 ml 0.2 M mercaptoethanol
 i. Sixteen 10-x-75-mm glass test tubes

2. Immunoglobulin Quantitation

 a. Commercially prepared immunodiffusion plates specific for one of the immunoglobulin classes
 b. Sera with known and unknown amounts of desired immunoglobulins
 c. If possible, sera from patients with known immunodeficiency or myeloma of the desired class
 d. Capillary pipettes
 e. Moist chambers
 f. 2-cycle semilogarithmic paper
 g. Viewer or microscope with ocular micrometer

EXERCISE 5: T-Cell and B-Cell Immunity

1. Enumeration of T- and B-cells

 a. Sterile 12-ml syringe with 1000 units of heparin or one heparinized Vacutainer and needle (Beckton, Dickenson and Company, Rutherford, NJ)
 b. Phosphate-buffered saline or Hanks Balanced Salt Solution (HBSS) (GIBCO, Grand Island, NY)
 c. Lymphocyte separation media (e.g., Ficol-Paque, Pharmacia Fine Chemicals, Piscataway, NJ)
 d. Sheep erythrocytes preserved in Alsever's solution or freshly drawn in heparin. Wash SRBCs 3X in saline, and resuspend to a 4×10^7/ml, approximately 0.1 ml packed cells in 5 ml saline.
 e. Immunobeads (Bio-Rad Laboratories, Rockville Centre, NY). Prepare the beads according to manufacturer's recommendations.
 f. 12-x-75-mm culture tubes (glass or plastic)
 g. Capillary pipettes
 h. Hemocytometer and cover slip

2. Demonstration of B-cell Dependent Function

 a. Control mice and mice previously immunized four days ahead of time (0.2 ml I. V. injection of 2% SRBCs per mouse) should be available.
 b. Sterile 9-cm Petri dishes
 c. Balanced salt solution (BSS):

KCl	0.45 g	
$MgSO_4 \cdot H_2O$	0.25 g	Adjust pH to 7.4 and
$CaCl_2$	0.22 g	sterilize by autoclaving
NaCl	7.01 g	
TRIS	1.21 g	
Distilled water	1000 ml	

 d. 100 ml 1% Noble's agar in BSS
 e. 100 ml 0.7% Noble's agar in BSS containing 50 mg DEAE-dextran

f.   Sterile scalpels, scissors, 2-ml syringes, and 20-gauge needles
g.   10 ml 10% SRBCs
h.   4 ml fresh guinea pig complement/plate diluted 1/7 with BSS

For the alternative method:

a.   Microscope slides
b.   Double-stick Scotch tape
c.   Molten wax or paraffin. It is best to use wax melted in a large Petri dish on a warming tray.

3.   Demonstration of T-cell Dependent Function

Tissue culture reagents required for this experiment can be purchased from a number of companies including GIBCO, M.A. Bioproducts, and Sigma.

a.   One mouse per group (This can be the control mouse from EXPERIMENT 2, if done on the same day.)
b.   Sterile scalpels, forceps, and scissors
c.   Hanks Balanced Salt Solution (HBSS), 50 ml per group
d.   Petri dishes, 60-mm size
e.   RPMI-1640 complete medium

RPMI-1640 with glutamine	90 ml
Fetal or newborn calf serum	10 ml
100X Pen-Strep Antibiotic Solution	1 ml
0.005 M 2-mercaptoethanol (Fisher)	1 ml

f.   Concanavalin A (Con A) (Sigma) dissolved in RPMI-1640 media to a final concentration of 1 to 5 μg/ml
g.   Phytohemagglutinin (PHA, e.g., Sigma's Leucoagglutinin, PHA-L) dissolved in RPMI-1640 to a final concentration of 5 to 10 μg/ml
h.   Humidified CO_2 incubator at 37°C. If a CO_2 incubator is not available, one can use any chamber flushed with 5% CO_2 in a conventional incubator.

EXERCISE 6: Agglutination

1.   Rapid Slide Agglutination

   a.   One agglutination slide per student
   b.   0.2 ml antiserum per student
   c.   Commercial slide agglutination antigens
   d.   0.2-ml pipettes
   e.   Applicator sticks

2.   Tube Agglutination

   a.   1 ml antiserum to any species of *Salmonella,* diluted 1/20
   b.   5 ml homologous antigen suspension (1 x 10^9 organisms/ml) per student
   c.   Ten 12-x-75-mm tubes per student

3.   Agglutinin Adsorption

   a.   1 ml 1/10 anti-*E. coli* 0127B8 serum per student of which anti-O and anti-B titers are known
   b.   1 ml of a heavy suspension of *E. coli* 0127B8 cells per pair of students
   c.   1 ml of a heavy suspension of *E. coli* 0127B8 cells previously heated 1 hr at 100°C per pair of students
   d.   5 ml *E. coli* 0127B8 cells (1 x 10^9 organisms/ml) per student
   e.   Twenty-two 12-x-75-mm tubes per student

4. Bacterial Inagglutinability

   a. 1 ml anti-*E. coli* 0127B8 diluted 1/20 per student
   b. 2.5 ml of a suspension (1 x 10^9 organisms/ml) of the homologous cells per student and a like amount of cells that have been heated 1 hr at 100°C
   c. Twenty 12-x-75-mm tubes per student

EXERCISE 7: Isoimmunization

1. Blood Typing (ABO)

   a. Unknown 5% human erythrocyte suspensions
   b. Commercial anti-A and anti-B typing sera
   c. Unknown human sera
   d. Known 5% suspensions of human A and B red cells
   e. Applicator sticks
   f. Microscope slides
   g. Sterile blood lancets, cotton pledgets, and 70% ethyl alcohol

2. Titration and Adsorption of O Serum

   a. 1 ml O serum per student
   b. 5 ml 2% suspension of A-cells per student
   c. 5 ml 2% suspension of B-cells per student
   d. 0.5 ml packed thrice-washed A- or B-cells per student
   e. Twenty 12-x-75-mm tubes per student

3. Compatibility Test—Direct Matching

   a. 0.5 ml donor's serum per student per test
   b. 0.5 ml recipient's serum per student per test
   c. 0.3 ml 3% donor's cells per student per test
   d. 0.3 ml 3% recipient's cells per student per test
   e. Six 12-x-75-mm tubes per student per test

4. Rh Tube Test

   a. Unknown saline suspensions (2%) of human erythrocytes
   b. Commercial typing sera
   c. 12-x-75-mm tubes
   d. Sterile lancets, cotton pledgets, and 70% alcohol

5. Rh Antibodies

   Blocking Test
   a. Four 12-x-75-mm tubes per student
   b. Two drops *slide/tube test* serum (anti-D) per student
   c. Four drops 2% saline suspension of D+ cells per student
   d. Four drops 2% saline suspension of D- cells per student
   e. Two drops saline agglutinating serum (anti-D) per student

   Coombs Test
   a. Four 12-x-75-mm tubes per student
   b. Two drops *slide/tube test* serum (anti-D) per student
   c. Four drops 2% saline suspension of D+ cells per student
   d. Four drops 2% saline suspension of D- cells per student
   e. Four drops Coombs serum per student

Protein Diluent Test
a.   Four drops 2% D+ cells suspended in 22% bovine albumin per student
b.   One drop 22% bovine albumin per student
c.   Two 12-x-75-mm tubes per student

Trypsinized Cell Technique
a.   1 ml 2% trypsinized D+ cells in saline per student (1 ml packed cells to 1.5 ml 0.1% trypsin-Difco 1:250; incubate at 37°C/30 min; wash three times
b.   0.1 ml *slide/tube test* serum (anti-D) per student
c.   Ten 12-x-75-mm tubes per student

EXERCISE 8: Microbial Hemagglutination

1.   Direct—Viral Hemagglutination and Hemagglutination Inhibition

   a.   Influenza virus—type A from EXERCISE 2, 2
   b.   15 ml 0.25% suspension of chicken erythrocytes per student
   c.   0.5 ml anti-influenza serum per student
   d.   Twenty-four 12-x-75-mm tubes per student
   e.   15 ml phosphate-buffered saline (pH 7.4) per student
   5.6 g Na_2HPO_4/liter
   2.7 g KH_2PO_4/liter
   4.1 g NaCl/liter

2.   Indirect Hemagglutination

   a.   1 ml washed packed sheep RBCs in 0.9% NaCl (Do *not* use phosphate-buffered saline.) Enough for ten batches
   b.   Freshly prepared 0.1% $CrCl_3$
   c.   0.1 ml human globulin at 0.5 mg/ml per batch
   d.   0.2 ml anti-human globulin diluted 1/20 per titration
   e.   Round bottom 10-x-75-mm serological tubes or microtiter equipment

EXERCISE 9: Precipitation

1.   Precipitin Analysis

Each student will need:

   a.   2 ml 0.05% ovalbumin or human serum albumin
   b.   6 ml homologous antiserum diluted 1/5 (clarify by filtration, if necessary)
   c.   Six heavy-walled centrifuge tubes (12 ml)
   d.   Twelve 12-x-75-mm tubes
   e.   3 ml antiserum 1/5
   f.   3 ml antigen diluted to equivalence (instructor must predetermine)
   g.   65 ml 2% $NaCO_3$ in 0.1 N NaOH
   h.   Six 16-x-100-mm test tubes
   i.   A seventh 16-x-100-mm tube containing 250 μg/ml rabbit globulin for use as a protein standard
   j.   75 ml alkaline tartrate solution
         50 parts 2% $NaCO_3$ in 0.1 N NaOH
           1 part 0.5% $CuSO_4$
           1 part 1% NaK Tartrate

Reagents must be added in order, slowly, with mixing between each step

k.   4 ml phenol reagent diluted 1/2 (e.g., Fisher Scientific Co., No. So-P-24)

l.   Vortex mixer and spectrophotometer/colorimeter at 660 μm

2. Gel Diffusion Analysis

a.   20 ml gel diffusion agar per student

  (1) Buffer solution

TRIS	0.93 g
sodium chloride	0.7 g
1 N HCl	7 to 8 ml to pH 7.4
distilled water	q.s. ad 100 ml

  (2) To every 100 ml of buffer, add 0.8 g agarose. Melt and pour 6 ml per 60-x-15-mm Petri dish

b.   Three 60-x-15-mm Petri dishes with diffusion agar per student

c.   Gel cutter

d.   Pasteur or capillary pipettes

e.   0.3 ml anti-bovine serum per student

f.   Log dilutions of bovine serum (0.3 ml each dilution per student)

g.   0.6 ml anti-human serum per student

h.   0.3 ml each human globulin and human albumin (1 mg/ml) per student

i.   Log dilutions of human serum (0.6 ml each dilution per student)

j.   Log dilutions of monkey serum (0.3 ml each dilution per student)

EXERCISE 10: Complement Fixation

NOTE: All reagents in this exercise should be prepared with saline to which $MgSO_4$ (0.1 g/liter) has been added. Veronal buffered saline is preferred. See EXPERIMENT 5.

1. Standardization of Components of the Indicator System

Titration of Hemolysin

a.   Twelve 13-x-100-mm tubes per student

b.   5 ml 1/1000 hemolysin per student

c.   30 ml Mag saline per student

d.   3.5 ml 1/30 pooled guinea pig complement per student

e.   6 ml 2% sheep erythrocyte suspension per student

Titration of Complement

a.   Eleven 13-x-100-mm test tubes per student

b.   3.5 ml 1/30 complement per student

c.   Optional: 5 ml of the appropriate dilution of antigen per student

d.   5 ml hemolysin (2 units per 0.5 ml) per student

e.   20 ml Mag saline per student

f.   6 ml 2% sheep cells per student

3. Determination of Antigenic Dose

a.   6.5 ml antigen in initial dilution per student

b.   4 ml known strongly positive serum 1/5 per student (freshly inactivated)

c.   33 ml complement (2 full units/ml) per student

d.   17 ml hemolysin (2 units/0.5 ml) per student

e.   17 ml 2% sheep cells per student

f.   Thirty-three 13-x-100-mm test tubes per student

4. Wassermann-Kolmer Test

    a. 0.4 ml each unknown antiserum per student
    b. 0.4 ml known positive serum per student
    c. 0.4 ml known negative serum per student

NOTE: All sera should be freshly inactivated ($56°C/30$ min).

    d. 2 ml of the appropriate dose of antigen per test per student
    e. 9 ml complement (2 full units/ml) per test per student
    f. 10 ml Mag saline per test per student
    g. 5 ml hemolysin (2 units/0.5 ml) per test per student
    h. 6 ml 2% sheep cells per test per student
    i. Eleven 13-x-100-mm test tubes per test per student

5. CH_{50} Determination

The use of barbiturates in veronal buffered saline may cause problems since these materials are controlled substances subject to regulation by the Federal Drug Enforcement Agency. If obtaining a federal permit just to obtain these materials is inconvenient, triethanolamine buffered saline (TBS) may be used instead.

    a. Triethanolamine buffered saline (TBS) 10 x stock with metals (Me^{++})

NaCl	150 g
Triethanolamine	56 ml
1 N HCl	324 ml
Stock metals solution	20 ml

($CaCl_2 \cdot 6H_2O$ - 16.4 g and $MgCl_2 \cdot 6H_2O$ 101.7 g dissolved in 500 ml distilled H_2O)

Distilled water   q.s. ad 2000 ml

Dilute 1/10 for use fresh daily, adding 10 ml 2.5% gelatin per liter as a stabilizer. Adjust pH to 7.3 to 7.4.

    b. 10 x TBS without metals
    c. 0.01 M EDTA-TBS buffer—make fresh each day
    20 ml 10 x TBS without Me^{++}
    13.3 ml 0.15 M Na_2 EDTA
    q.s. ad to 200 ml
    d. 5 ml SRBCs in Alsever's solution/group
    e. Commercial anti-sheep erythrocyte serum (hemolysin)
    f. Colorimeter capable of reading in the 412 to 541 mμ ranges
    g. 0.1 ml fresh human or 0.2 ml fresh rabbit serum per determination

6. The Alternative Pathway

    a. It is suggested that this experiment be done by small groups of students
    b. 2 ml fresh guinea pig, human, or rabbit serum per group
    c. 0.3 ml 1% inulin per group
    d. 25 μl 0.1 M disodium EDTA per group
    e. 25 μl MgEGTA per group. Suspend EGTA (Sigma Chemical Co., St. Louis, MO) at 0.1 M and 70 mM $MgCl_2 \cdot 6H_2O$ in saline. Dissolve at $60°C$ and add 5 N NaOH until material just goes into solution. Add more NaOH until pH 7.3.
    f. Saline
    g. 80 μl 0.1 M Ca_2Cl_2 per group
    h. VBS and sensitized SRBCs as in previous experiment; enough for four determinations per group

EXERCISE 11: ELISA

1. Coating Buffer

Na_2CO_3	3.18 g
$NaHCO_3$	5.84 g
Distilled water	1000 ml
Adjust pH to	9.5

2. Diluting Buffer

(A) 0.5 M KH_2PO_4	100 ml
(B) 0.5 M KH_2PO_4	30 ml
Tween 20	0.5 ml
NaCl	8.5 g
Distilled water	q.s. ad 1000 ml

    Adjust pH to 7.2; use Solution B to raise pH
    use Solution A to lower pH

3. Wash Buffer

    Same as step 2 only do not add Tween 20

4. Substrate Buffer

K_2HPO_4	11.85 g
Citric acid	11.73 g
Distilled water	q.s. ad 1000 ml
Adjust pH to	4.0

5. Substrate: dissolve 10 mg 2,2'-azino-di-(3-ethylbenzthiazoline sulfonic acid), diammonium salt (Sigma No. A-1888, St. Louis, MO) in 50 ml substrate buffer, and add 10 μl 30% H_2O_2. This must be made fresh each time.

6. 1.2 ml ovalbumin, 10 μg/ml dissolved in coating buffer, per student

7. 0.5 ml anti-ovalbumin diluted 1/50 in diluting buffer

8. Ten 12-x-75-mm tubes per student

9. 1.3 ml commercial goat anti-rabbit globulin conjugated to horseradish peroxidase, per student. Dilute to 1/500 in diluting buffer.

10. Plastic microtiter plates (e.g., Immunlon I, Dynatech Laboratories, Alexandria, VA), micro-pipettes or microdiluters, and small, humid chambers to prevent plates from drying out during incubation. An ELISA reader and multiwell plate washers would also be exceedingly useful.

EXERCISE 12: Gel Filtration

1. Desalting Precipitated Globulins

    These are the materials necessary for one run:

    a. 20 g G-25 Sephadex swelled at least 3 hr in 300 ml saline
    b. Glass column approximately 2.5 cm wide and 60 to 80 cm high
    c. One elution reservoir or separatory funnel
    d. Connection tubing for reservoir and column outflow

e. Screw clamp
f. Glass rod
g. Water aspirator for degassing slurry and saline
h. 5 ml serum
i. Ice bath
j. 10 ml saturated $(NH_4)_2SO_4$
k. 30 ml half-saturated $(NH_4)_2SO_4$
l. Ten 13-x-100-mm test tubes
m. One heavy-walled 12-ml centrifuge tube
n. Capillary pipettes
o. 10% $BaCl_2$ solution, if desired

2. Immunoglobulin Separation

a. 1.5-cm column containing G-200 Sephadex (allow 1 g resin to swell three days in 200 ml saline)
b. 0.5-ml serum sample containing IgM red cell agglutinins
c. Automatic fraction collector
d. Automatic ultraviolet absorption monitor or ultraviolet spectrophotometer
e. Immunoelectrophoresis equipment or materials to titrate versus specific red cells

EXERCISE 13: Chromatography

1. DEAE Ion Exchange Chromatography

These are the materials necessary for one run:

a. Solutions. Formulas for all the solutions needed are on page 77.

b. DEAE Cellulose

(1) 2 g DEAE cellulose
(2) 4 liters 0.5 M Na Cl
(3) 500 ml 0.1 M NaOH

c. Column

(1) One glass column 30 cm high and 1 cm I. D.
(2) One 100-ml beaker
(3) One 50-ml Erlenmeyer flask
(4) One magnetic stirrer
(5) One ring stand

d. Chromatography

(1) Serum sample containing 10 to 30 mg protein
(2) Capillary pipettes
(3) Rubber tubing
(4) Fraction collector and tubes
(5) Immunodiffusion equipment and/or ultraviolet spectrophotometer

2. Rapid Separation of IgM from IgG

a. One Quik-Sep IgM Isolation Column (System II) per student. Kits of 20 or 100 columns, including all necessary buffers, can be obtained from Isolab, Drawer 4350, Akron, OH 44321.
b. 0.2 ml anti-*Salmonella* serum (or any anti-Gram-negative coliform serum) per student
c. Suspension of homologous antigen diluted appropriately (see EXERCISE 6, 2)

EXERCISE 14: Electrophoresis

1. Cellulose Acetate Electrophoresis

   a. Formulae for solutions and stain appear with the experimental directions
   b. Commercial electrophoresis chamber suitable for cellulose acetate strips
   c. Cellulose acetate strips
   d. Protein-containing sample
   e. Micropipette, 2 μl

2. Immunoelectrophoresis

   a. Formulae for solutions and stain appear with the experimental directions
   b. Suitable electrophoresis apparatus
   c. Glass slides
   d. Sera or other suitable samples
   e. Suitable antisera
   f. Suitable agar cutters
   g. Capillary pipettes

EXERCISE 15: Immunohistochemistry

1. Immunofluorescence. In addition to the buffers described in the instructions, the following additional materials will be necessary:

   a. Gel-filtration apparatus and reagents for desalting (EXERCISE 12)
   b. Lowry protein reagents (EXERCISE 9) and spectrophotometer
   c. Smears of appropriate microorganisms
   d. Five staining dishes or Coplin jars
   e. 95% ethanol
   f. Capillary pipettes
   g. Cover slips
   h. Buffered glycerol (mix 9 parts glycerine with 1 part carbonate-bicarbonate buffer)
   i. An ultraviolet-illuminated microscope with dark field condenser, UV adsorbing eyepieces, and a 2- to 3- or 5-mm UV transmission filter

NOTE: If commercial antiglobulin is to be used, the titer may be unknown and it will be necessary to determine this using gel-diffusion plates.

EXERCISE 16: Immediate Hypersensitivity

1. Anaphylaxis

   a. Six 400- to 500-g guinea pigs per class
   b. 20 ml horse serum per class
   c. 1 ml high-titered anti-horse serum per class
   d. Sterile 2-ml syringes and 24-gauge needles
   e. Autopsy instruments

2. Passive Cutaneous Anaphylaxis

   a. Six 300- to 400-g guinea pigs
   b. Anti-bovine serum albumin, sterile, 1/20

    c.   Sterile 5% bovine serum albumin
    d.   1% Evans blue

3. Action of Histamine and Antihistamines

    a.   Two normal 400- to 500-g guinea pigs
    b.   Two horse-serum-hypersensitive guinea pigs
    c.   Benadryl (Parke, Davis and Co., Detroit, MI)
    d.   4 ml horse serum
    e.   Solution of histamine
    f.   Sterile syringes and needles

EXERCISE 17: Cytotoxic Reactions

1. Masugi Nephritis

    a.   Twenty rat kidneys
    b.   Sterile Waring blender
    c.   1 liter sterile phosphate-buffered saline
    d.   Vials of Freund's complete and incomplete adjuvant (Difco Laboratories, Detroit, MI)
    e.   Six rats and two to four rabbits
    f.   50-50 ethanol ether
    g.   95% ethanol
    h.   Fluorescein-conjugated anti-rabbit globulin 1/20 and appropriate FA reagents

EXERCISE 18: Immune Complex Reactions

1. The Arthus Reaction

    a.   1% ovalbumin
    b.   One rabbit

2. Glomerulonephritis

These are the materials necessary for one group of experimental animals:

    a.   Three 2-kg rabbits
    b.   10 ml 1% bovine serum albumin
    c.   Materials for precipitin, supernate, and pricipitate analyses (see EXERCISE 9)
    d.   Commercially labeled fluorescent antiserum to rabbit globulin and bovine serum albumin
    e.   Dissecting instruments
    f.   Other materials necessary for fluorescent microscopy
    g.   Normal, fresh or frozen, rabbit kidney
    h.   Immunization syringes

EXERCISE 19: Cell-Mediated Reactions

1. Delayed Hypersensitivity

    a.   Allergy of Infection. These are the materials necessary per guinea pig:
        (1) Depilatory agent

      (2) 0.5 ml Freund's complete adjuvant containing TB bacilli (Difco Laboratories, Detroit, MI)

      (3) 0.1 PPD, Second Strength (Parke, Davis and Co., Detroit, MI)

  b. Contact Dermatitis

    (1) Control guinea pigs
      (a) 3 ml absolute ethanol
      (b) Glass rod

    (2) Test guinea pigs
      (a) 3 ml 2% 2,4-dinitrochlorobenzene (DNCB) in absolute ethanol
      (b) Glass rod

2. Migration Inhibition Factor (MIF)

  a. Specialized Glassware

    (1) Diffusion chamber. This technique will require the use of special plastic diffusion chambers (Mackaness chambers, Berton Plastics, South Hackensack, NJ). These are essentially thick microscope slides with a special chamber drilled in the middle of each. Prepare the chambers by boiling for 10 min in 1% trichloracetic acid (TCA); wash with tissue-culture grade detergent; rinse several times in tap water, once in distilled water, once in isopropanol, and wipe dry. Place on gauze in Petri dishes, and sterilize in an autoclave.

    (2) Capillary tubes and cover slips. Wash capillary tubes (1.1- to 1.2-mm I. D.) in distilled water only. Cover slips (22-mm circular) are prepared in the same manner as the chambers, omitting only the boiling in TCA. Tubes and cover slips are then placed in Petri dishes and sterilized in a dry-air oven 4 to 5 hr.

    (3) Assembly of chambers. Immediately after autoclaving chambers, place one cover slip over hole in chamber and seal with hot paraffin. Invert chamber, and place a small dot of sterile silicone grease on the cover slip just above the two entry ports. Store in a sterile, dust-free container.

    (4) Cell harvesting tube. This is prepared by perforating a 16-x-125-mm plastic, screw-top tissue-culture tube (Falcon Plastics, Oxnard, CA) with a hot 18-gauge needle. Keep sterile during and after perforation.

  b. Other materials (for each guinea pig):

    (1) 20 to 25 ml sterile mineral oil
    (2) 30-ml sterile glass syringe with 15-gauge needle
    (3) Ether or other suitable anesthesia
    (4) Dissection kit including two hemostats
    (5) Two ring stands fitted with cross bar
    (6) 120 ml Hanks balanced salt solution (HBSS)
    (7) 35 ml heparinized HBSS (500 units/ml)
    (8) Three sterile 50-ml screw-cap centrifuge tubes
    (9) Two sterile 10-ml screw-cap centrifuge tubes
    (10) Suitable antigens. PPD (Parke, Davis and Co., Detroit, MI) and/or heterologous protein antigen
    (11) Hematocrit centrifuge
    (12) Swinging bucket centrifuge for each type of centrifuge tube
    (13) Tuberculin syringes with 27-gauge needles
    (14) Additional hot paraffin
    (15) Viewing screen attachment for microscope
    (16) Planimeter (desired but optional)
    (17) Gaseous CO_2

(18) Aqueous sodium bicarbonate, tissue-culture grade 5.6% (Flow Laboratories, Inc., Rockville, MD)

(19) Additional Hanks minimal essential medium (MEM) with 15% normal guinea pig serum

3. Auto-immunity—Allergic Encephalomyelitis

    a. Sterile phosphate-buffered saline
    b. Freund's complete adjuvant (Difco Laboratories, Detroit, MI)
    c. Sterile syringe fitted with short 20-gauge needle
    d. Dissection equipment
    e. Ether or other suitable anesthesia
    f. Sterile 1-ml syringes
    g. Guinea pigs (300 to 350 q)

NOTE: The brain-spinal cord extract from one guinea pig will produce enough antigen for the injection of three to four guinea pigs.

FURTHER SUGGESTIONS FOR INSTRUCTOR OR ASSISTANTS

Some of the experiments call for materials only available from hospitals or medical centers, which may tend to complicate preparing some of the experiments for those attempting to teach immunology in a nonmedical institution. This disadvantage is easily overcome in the authors' experience by utilizing various community sources of supply. Blood banks at hospitals are usually very cooperative in supplying human erythrocytes from outdated blood donations. They may also be able to supply outdated typing sera. Sheep blood may be purchased through any number of laboratory supply houses, while local veterinarians have proven helpful in supplying blood samples from a number of domestic animals.

Often patient material may be obtained from the clinical laboratories of community hospitals, and some companies even offer certain types of pathologic sera for control purposes (Wassermann reactive sera, myeloma sera, etc.). Pharmacists at drug stores have proven helpful in obtaining certain materials such as diphtheria antitoxin and similar biological pharmaceuticals.

Since this manual was begun at a nonmedical school, the authors are particularly sensitive to the ease of obtaining teaching materials and offer their assistance to instructors having difficulty locating supplies.